IRREVOCABLE

T. E. Shaw

authorHOUSE®

AuthorHouse™ UK Ltd.
500 Avebury Boulevard
Central Milton Keynes, MK9 2BE
www.authorhouse.co.uk
Phone: 08001974150

First published by AuthorHouse 12/15/2009

ISBN: 978-1-4490-5836-4 (e)
ISBN: 978-1-4490-5837-1 (sc)

This book is printed on acid-free paper.

PROLOGUE.

I had been having this recurring dream every night for the past week and it was really starting to make me wonder.

The scene was set in what must have been a church. Everything was white; a vision of purity.

I was being walked down the aisle, dressed in a fine black suit, my dad at one side and Nana on my arm. Everyone was smiling up at me as I moved by, and I realised after a time that I was smiling, too. The dream always started out well, even though, initially, I didn't think to question where it might lead.

The aisle was long, and the pews either side of me were full, though I didn't recognise any of the faces. As we moved on, I looked ahead to see, standing at the front of the church, a minister and my two favourite people - Zen and Frankie - waiting eagerly for me with broad, sincere smiles reaching from cheek to cheek. However, there was one other person there, and they had their back to me.

They were wearing a black suit almost identical to mine, and I was curious to know who they were. Why weren't they looking at me like everyone else?

Although not a hundred percent sure why we were even here to begin with, I still had an inkling. But being that it *was* a dream, I just figured that anything could happen anywhere. And yet, if this dream was, in fact, going in the very direction I thought it was, shouldn't there be an elegant woman in white somewhere? I wouldn't linger too long on that thought, however, as the mystery of the person in black was really starting to bug me. While they appeared to be as much of a stranger to me as the rest of the spectators around me, something about them lured me in. I couldn't put my finger on it, but I had to know who *they* were, at least, if no-one else.

Once we had reached the front, the minister - a large, jolly-looking woman with dark, cropped hair - grinned warmly and held out her arms to welcome me.

As Dad and Nana found their seats, I positioned myself in front of said minister, though not without keeping a probing eye on the stranger beside me. Even right up close to them as I was now, I still couldn't see their face. This was mainly because they didn't actually seem to have a one. It was as if their hair had deliberately grown out to conceal it, keeping me in suspense for just that extra bit longer.

'You may now kiss the groom,' the minister sang.

Oh? That's funny, I hadn't even said 'I do,' yet...And groom? Shouldn't it be bride?...Where *was she*, anyway?

The reality then dawned on me: there was *no* bride. I couldn't object to anything, though; I no longer had a voice. I felt like an old silent movie character misplaced in a talky.

The faceless, shaggy thing slowly began to turn towards me - was *this* what I had married? As they did, their hair started to fall away, steadily revealing more human-like flesh - at least it *was* human! It looked down, and the last of the covering hair fell to the ground. It then looked back up at me and blinded me at once with heart-stopping radiance.

At that precise moment, however, the subconsciously constructed image would immediately fade and I would wake up, tormented by confusion.

I never did remember who it was that was so blinding. Until one day, when I kind of got an inkling.

CHAPTER 1.

I let the tepid water trickle over my hands until I was satisfied they were clean enough.

Friday 4th September - the first day back at school after a somewhat uneventful summer holiday, and it was break time.

I inhaled deeply, blinking back the sleep in my eyes from my recent disturbed nights. I then exhaled. Back to school again, the seemingly endless cycle of education continuing. I mean, you go away for six weeks, and then when you come back, you find life almost exactly the way you left it. Just maybe a little harder and with a few new faces. It was the same every year - boring.

I was in my last year at Audley Upper, so of course I was hearing no end of the dreaded GCSE's. I would no doubt also be expected to consider starting my revision as soon as possible, even though we hadn't really learnt anything new yet and the final exams were virtually a whole year off. But, as per usual, that didn't stop me from worrying myself stupid over how I would fair at the end of it all. Typical me.

The toilets were busy. Lads came and went, bringing with them noise and loutish friends. I wanted to get out of there quickly before anyone I knew and didn't like decided to put in an appearance. That was the thing about high school, unless you were one of the coolest of the cool, you would always be subject to passing pranks and childish name calling. Degrading, really, but then that's school social politics for you.

Just as I was about to move away from the basin to the hand dryers, out of the corner of my eye, I absentmindedly noticed someone had come up to the one beside me. On further, brief, inspection, I managed to deduce that the guy, decked out in dark blue denim jeans and a stripy black and white rugby shirt, was a sixth former.

He was having trouble working the infamously fiddly taps, as the water was exploding everywhere. This guy was also obviously a newbie, because anyone who had been at the school long enough would have known by now that to get these taps to cooperate, you had to press down on them gently. Fortunately for him, not many people had seen this slightly embarrassing spectacle. And, feeling charitable for no particular reason - but also trying not to make it seem as though I had seen too much - I subtly went through the motions of how it should be done. He must have picked up on my little hint, because without saying a word, he did as I did, and this time the tap behaved. I turned to face him. He looked up in relief and nodded a 'thank you' before moving to leave.

With that fleeting look of acknowledgment, came a well timed, sharp punch from somewhere deep in my gut. Though I knew I had never laid eyes on this guy before, something inside me screamed at a sense of familiarity.

His face was wide and handsome; his light brown hair was short and neatly gelled into a trendy little coif at the front, and his eyes were a captivatingly steely blue. He was a little shorter than me, but more filled out - stocky, but also lightly toned. He really was quite impressive to look at, and I almost felt unworthy in his presence.

The bell rang out, signalling the end of break and the beginning of third period. I felt a little dazed and suddenly sore in the chest. Maybe it was just Nana's own rendition of a fry-up from earlier that was making me feel so weird. She wasn't used to doing much and had attempted to cook breakfast for a change. Bless her heart, though, she was hardly a Nigella Lawson in the kitchen.

I sat through the whole of Maths really not concentrating at all. It was the first day back, though, so I guessed it was only to be expected. Not helped by the fact that Maths was also the bane of my existence!

I was starting to daydream in between fractions and thought back to before, in the toilets, about that guy I had seen. The image of him reappeared in my mind and I was intrigued; I wanted to know more about him. I tried to envision what he was like as a person, wondering what he studied. Being a sixth former, I bet he didn't do Maths anymore. No, he looked much too cool for that. I mean, not even *I* would be caught dead carrying a Maths text book once the GCSE's were over, and I'm what's colourfully described as a "boff." Anyway, only truly mad people, like prospective teachers, took Maths on further than they actually had to. No, my guess was that this guy obviously studied something along the lines of P.E. - among other things, of course. Sure enough, he looked like he would be good at sports. You would have to be with a physique like his. I bet the girls went all goo-goo eyed when they saw him out in his kit on the pitch. Though I hated sports altogether, should I ever have the urge to watch a school match of some kind involving him, I bet he would be quite a player to look out for.

Lunchtime, and food was the last thing on my mind. Zen and Frankie weren't impressed by my vacant expressions and long silences, either.

'Yo! Wake up, dude!' Frankie crowed in my ear, snapping her fingers as if to dehypnotise me.

'Yeah, you're dead to the world, mate. It's lunchtime, for Christ's sake!' Zen added with a mouthful of ham and cheese. 'Eat up!'

My own sandwiches lay in front of me on the table wrapped in Clingfilm, looking sad and unwanted. I didn't care, though. I really didn't feel much like eating right now; there was too much on my mind. I was having a very strange day today in general, and didn't exactly feel like my old self. But whatever the matter was, I was still letting myself believe that it was all just first-day-back blues.

'Sorry guys. You know what, I'm gonna save this for later. Maybe my appetite will have come back by then,' I reasoned, pushing the untouched lunch back into my bag.

Still the odd feelings would not go away all day, and I felt constantly agitated. I thought that maybe I was just a little under the weather, as I was certainly never one to turn down food.

Come fifth period, I asked to be excused from class so that I could visit the sick bay. I thought it would be better to be sure than to leave things. This was, after all, one of the strangest sensations I had ever had. Miss Rook, my English teacher, said she thought I looked fine, but that she trusted me enough to let me go. Though not before being jeered out of the room by my envious fellow peers, of course - the privileges of being a "boff," I suppose.

'Well, you look fine to me, dearie,' said the sick bay nurse, smiling patronisingly. 'Whatever it is you think you're feeling might have something to do with your hormones. Or indeed, you might have just eaten something a little *offish*.'

'Hmph, that's reassuring,' I muttered sarcastically under my breath. Hormones are a teenager's worst nightmare and I was no exception. I felt I knew myself enough, though, to not go along with that prognosis. So, instead, I was going to go with dodgy food as the culprit for my body's sudden upturn. I didn't usually get tummy bugs, so that may well have been all it was. The weirdest thing was that these strange sensations had only really started up after my trip to the loo at break time, after I had bumped into *him*...whoever *he* was. Maybe it was just some bizarre coincidence.

Anyway, it was nearing the end of the day, and once I got back home I would be able to lie down for a while to clear my head.

CHAPTER 2.

Greville Rd. was where I lived with my dad and Nana; we ran a B&B together. The Brambles, it was called - right bang-smack in the middle of the typically picturesque Suffolk village of Hobden.

Well, I say *we*, but it really was mainly my dad who ran the family business. Not exactly the manliest of men, Dad was definitely a house proud wizard. He could cook anything, and cleaned everything until it glistened. The B&B was everything to him and it reflected on him so well. Nana, on the other hand, did what she could as and when, but she suffered from chronic arthritis, and there were often days at a time when she couldn't do much of anything because of the pain. She never spoke much, either - not since my mum died a few years back. I guess no parent should have to bury their own child, or so the saying goes, and she had never quite been the same since.

As I walked up the mossy garden path to our small, red-bricked, Edwardian country house, I kicked myself for having forgotten that we were expecting new guests that evening. I wasn't in the mood for more strangers in my home - not tonight, anyway. One of the major drawbacks for a teenager living in a working home is that you never really get much time to yourself. It would also mean that I would be expected to help Dad by making the new guests feel welcome, and of course, be on my "best behaviour." I didn't need the hassle today, really. I just wanted to be left well alone.

I quietly let myself into the narrow, tile-floored lobby and hurried up the rickety flight of stairs to my room, hoping that Dad hadn't noticed and that I would be able to hide away for at least a half an hour.

Opening the door to my room, head slumped, I tutted at myself for remembering I hadn't locked it that morning before school. I wasn't doing well today.

'Oh, hey!'

I half jumped out of my skin. Someone was in my room!…I shouldn't have been all that surprised, really, as it had happened before when I had forgotten to lock up. But this person was alarmingly familiar, and he was sitting right at the foot of my bed, unpacking a large holdall.

'Sorry, have I got the wrong room?' he asked, looking about him in confusion.

My throat went dry and my eyes went wide with disbelief. It was that really cool guy I had helped out with the tap situation in the toilets that morning at break!

Just hearing those very words circling around my head made me feel instantly ridiculous, but my tummy was doing funny summersaults all the same, and the heavy pounding in my chest felt as though it would crack through my ribs.

'Erm, yeah. Sorry, yes, I'm, err, afraid you have, actually,' I stuttered and guffawed nervously. The stranger on my bed gave an amused chuckle in return. I felt my cheeks go bright red with embarrassment. Damn, I hate my laugh! It's so weird, and it makes people laugh at me.

'Must admit, I did think it looked a little too done up in here for a guest's bedroom. I'm Dean, by the way.' He smiled emphatically, then narrowed his eyes at me. 'You know, I'm sure I recognise you from somewhere…'

So he remembered me, too!…Sort of.

'Y-yeah, I remember. From school today. Though only very briefly, mind.'

I couldn't bloody well not remember him!

I was still reeling from the initial shock of the situation. But, my God, he really was quite remarkable to look at. I was even getting a little hot under the collar…Bloody hell! Why *was* it so hot all of a sudden?!

'So you're one of our Mackellar guests, then?' I blurted out, trying, rather unsuccessfully, to act unperturbed and as if I hadn't just suffered a minor stroke.

'Yip. Just me and my mum. We're only here for a little while, though. You know, just 'til we get a place of our own,' he said, looking me over and smiling again - most likely at the pathetic look on my face, but it was an infectious smile, nonetheless. 'So, erm, you must be Laurence, right?'

'Right, yes, Laurence...or, or just plain *Loz*. Either way.' I shrugged stupidly.

'Well, nice to meet you, Loz.' He held out a firm-looking hand for me to shake. I took it, slightly hesitant. My palms were clammy and my heart beat even faster at the touch of his flesh. He had a rough grip.

'Right. Well, I'm gonna go try and find my own room now, mate. Doesn't look too good when you make yourself at home in the wrong parts of a house that isn't yours,' he said jovially, getting up and moving towards the door with his bag slung over one shoulder. I went all tingly as he brushed past me. 'I'm sure my room's around here somewhere...'

Instinctively, I jumped at the chance to help.

'Did you want me to show you where it is?...I mean, I had to set it up this morning before school,...so I know which room it is.' I stopped briefly, slightly taken aback by my own forwardness. 'That is...if you want me to,...that is?'

His impressive eyes twinkled at me and he grinned. Though he was probably trying to suppress laughter at how much of an idiot I was evidently making of myself. I mean, how many times did the word *is* need to be repeated in any one sentence, exactly?

I was definitely feeling out of sorts, and must have looked like a complete pillock, gawping as I did. I almost hoped he would tell me what he thought was wrong with me, because honest to God, I certainly didn't...or at least I certainly didn't like to think why.

'Sounds like a plan!' he eventually agreed. 'Lead the way.'

Dean's room was actually only across the hall from mine. This made me feel even more of a dunce, because I could have easily just told him that rather than shown him, but he didn't seem to mind, and appreciated the help all the same. So I left him to get on with his unpacking.

I rushed back to my own room, a little distressed by what had just happened and how I had behaved in the last five minutes. There was a lot to process in my head, and I was a bit worried to say the least. What was it about him that had made me act so strangely? I know I hadn't exactly expected to find him in my own home, but even shocks like that didn't normally make you feel such a combination of giddiness and anticipation, did they? His being here was definitely a peculiar coincidence, given that I had been subconsciously thinking about him all day, as well.

With that thought in mind, and practically choking on my own breath, I then wondered whether or not I had a little crush on Dean. I had certainly never felt like that before about anyone else…No, I couldn't have a crush on him. I had just met the guy! And anyway, I wasn't gay. I mean, I had never really liked any of the girls at my school, but that didn't mean I liked the guys any more so. I just must strongly idolise Dean, that's all. Yes, I was sure that was all it was, idolism. He just simply was very cool, incredibly handsome and maybe someone to aspire to. This was a possibility that was far easier to accept than the alternative, at any rate.

By dinnertime, Dad had found me and forced me to help him dish up. Steak, chips and peas. My least favourite, seeing as I hated chips, I hated peas and I really wasn't that keen on any kind of meat that wasn't chicken. Still, I suppose you cater for the masses, right?

At least I got to meet Mrs Mackellar, who was eagerly awaiting her dinner at the dining room table. And who, might I add, looked almost absolutely nothing like her son. She was tall, painfully skinny, with red-brown hair and tired eyes hidden behind ridiculous librarian-style specs. She seemed friendly enough, though, and her small mouth would always curl up into a warm smile at the sight of me coming in and out of the kitchen with the plates and condiments.

'So, you're in your last year of secondary school, I hear, Laurence,' Mrs Mackellar confirmed in her best upper-middle class accent, as I placed Nana's already dished up plate of food in front of her and sat down beside her to help her cut it up - her arthritic hands were especially bad this evening. 'Big year ahead, then, eh?'

'Yes, I suppose,' I answered politely, while fighting my way through a tough bit of gristle. 'Can hardly say I'm looking forward to it, though, if I'm honest.'

'No, of course not. Nasty year all round, I'm afraid. Still, I'm sure you'll do well. You seem like a bright lad to me.'

'Thank you, Mrs Mackellar.'

How I hated ass-kissing idle chitchat!

'Bonnie, please, dear…My Goodness! Where on Earth is that boy of mine? I told him dinner was ready ages ago! It'll all go cold if he's not careful…Ah! Here he comes. I assume you two have met already?' Bonnie asked as her son entered the room. Something inside of me lurched forward again at the sight of him and it was really starting to get on my nerves.

'Hey, all!…Yeah, me and Loz, here, are well acquainted, aren't we? He showed me out of his room after I managed to get myself lost,' Dean tittered to himself, pulling up a chair next to his mother.

'Oh, honestly, Dean!…I'm so sorry about that, Laurence, dear. He's a bit deaf on instructions sometimes, this one,' Mrs Mackellar sighed, eye-balling her son. Dean shot an icy stare back at her.

'Well, Mr Price did tell you exactly where you needed to go, Dean!' she scolded.

This was so not worth a telling off, but then you often find that parents do that sometimes when they are around people they don't know very well; they try to demonstrate their parenting skills by belittling their kids in front of you. I felt quite sorry for Dean.

'It doesn't matter; don't worry about it,' I assured her, coming to his rescue, not liking to see him disempowered. I don't appreciate being in the middle of other people's arguments at the best of times, especially not at the dinner table - that's enough to put anyone off their food!

Thankfully, and not a moment too soon, Dad came in carrying a plate full of sliced, buttered bread and placed it in the middle of the table. He then waddled his way round to his seat.

'Ah, Dean! Nice to see you again. Help yourself to whatever you like, mate,' he cooed, as he spooned half a bowl-full of peas onto his own plate. 'There's more chips, as well, if anyone wants them.'

Dinner was slow. I kept eying Dean. Watching him eat was so strangely mesmerizing that I kept forgetting to eat my own food. Fortunately, I stopped myself each time before it became too obvious and someone ended up getting completely the wrong idea.

Meanwhile, Bonnie and Dad were totally engrossed in each other's company. Occasionally, though, they would call upon either me or Dean for feedback on the food, or to back them up on their stories.

Nana just sat at the end of the table, keeping herself to herself as always, smiling up at me every so often in gratitude for the little things I helped her with. But, each time I did lean over to help her, I could swear I felt a certain pair of eyes following my every move. I daren't look up to see if it was who I secretly hoped it was, and so just put it to the back of my mind as a silly paranoid thought and carried on eating.

'Oh, by the way, Loz,' Dad called down the table to me. 'Mrs Mac...*Bonnie*...wanted to know if you'd wait up for Dean tomorrow morning and make your way to the school bus stop together?'

I gulped silently and replied, if somewhat wobbly, 'Yeah, sure. No worries.' This might prove to be interesting.

'Cheers, mate,' said Dean, between mouthfuls.

'Yes, thank you, dear,' Bonnie added appreciatively, before turning back to her son to mouth something that looked a lot like 'slow down.' Dean just rolled his eyes up to heaven, and I stifled a laugh; his expressions were quite humorous sometimes.

After dessert, Dad and I cleared everything away into the kitchen and started to wash up. Both our guests had offered to do it themselves, but Dad wouldn't hear of it. Instead, he shimmied both them and Nana into the sitting room, made them a fire and showed them how to work the telly. Nana just fell asleep in her old, worn out chair and pouf in the corner.

'So, how was your first day back, matey?' Dad asked, his hands in the Marigolds and deep in suds.

'Yeah, alright, I guess.'

I wasn't in the mood for talking much at the moment. I just wanted to get the drying up done and go back up to my room. I didn't care whether this made me antisocial, I was not feeling at all like my old self today and hoped that some time to myself, or maybe even a good night's sleep, would do the trick and put me to right.

'Just "alright?"'

'Uh-huh,' I grunted back, hoping he would take the hint.

'Sure there isn't anything else you want to tell me?' he persisted.

Typical parent! Why couldn't he just let it lie?

'It went fine, Dad. Just fine!' I snapped.

'*O*-kay…Sorry I asked, then,' he retaliated.

I felt instantly guilty. 'Look, I'm sorry. I'm feeling a little *off* at the moment, but it's probably just because I'm tired.' Silence. 'I think I'm gonna head up to bed soon, anyway.'

'Ha! A teenager going to bed early?! Never thought I'd see the day!' Dad gloated light-heartedly.

I smirked and punched him playfully on the arm.

'Anyway, on a completely unrelated note…What do you think of our new tenants?'

'They're okay. But how long are they staying with us, again?' I asked, surprisingly genuinely interested.

'About two and a half months. Or at least until Bonnie can find them somewhere more permanent. It's not been an easy move for them, you know, coming up from down London way and moving all the way out in the sticks. Still, when those generous job offers come through, you've got to go where the money's at. Good thing is, at least we'll have some stable income for a while.'

'Hmm,' I agreed. 'So, what does Mrs Mackellar do, again?'

'That I'm not too sure of. Something to do with gas engineering, I think. She seems very nice, though, doesn't she?' He turned to me in earnest.

'Oh, yeah, definitely!' I smiled. I could tell he secretly liked her more than he was letting on. It had been embarrassingly obvious throughout the entire meal. Dad tended to babble a lot whenever he got talking to someone he really liked. For Bonnie Mackellar, however, it had proved to be a pretty endearing trait, as she giggled away flirtatiously, and rather tiresomely, at virtually everything he had had to say.

There was more silence for a few moments.

'And what about Dean? Nice young chap, isn't he? Think he's about a year or two older than you, actually,' Dad continued.

'Uh-huh, yeah, he's in the sixth form,' I mumbled. I didn't feel at all comfortable talking about Dean in front of Dad. Luckily, I had just finished drying up, and so hastily said goodnight - accidentally on purpose forgetting to say anything to Dean and his mum - and went upstairs to shower and go to bed. Today had been quite a day and right now I really needed to disconnect. Tomorrow would be a new day, a different day…perhaps.

That night, my recurring dream didn't come back. In fact, from then on, it never did.

CHAPTER 3.

7:00am sharp the next morning, and my alarm was ringing away annoyingly in my ear beside me on the bedside table. Normally, I would clumsily whack the snooze button and roll back over to grab a few extra sneaky minutes of sleep. But today, something was forcing me to get up that little bit earlier.

Due to my sleepiness, I couldn't quite remember why, but I just knew I had something very important to do this morning. I lay and wondered at first whether yesterday hadn't all just been a dream, a frustrating, yet slightly curious dream. But I knew instantly that it hadn't been. It had all seemed far too real...

At last, I remembered what it was I was supposed to be doing. I was supposed to be showing Dean to the school bus stop. I smiled automatically to myself; I was showing potentially the coolest and most good-looking guy in school to the bus stop. Then I fell into a fit of nervousness. I was showing potentially the coolest and most good-looking guy in school to the bus stop! I couldn't mess this up, Dean would be counting on me! I didn't want to look like a total spaz standing next to him, and I certainly didn't want people thinking, 'who's that spaz walking around with that really cool guy over there?' I wanted to look and feel like I deserved Dean's acknowledgement.

I dragged myself like a Neanderthal over to the basin in the corner of my room, which Dad had put in especially to stop me from being so late for school in the mornings due to my having to wait ages for our guests to finish up first in the main bathrooms.

I looked into the little mirror hung above the sink and cringed at what I saw. It was not a pretty sight. Not only did I look like a constellation, with spots dotted around my face, but my dark hair stuck up all over, doing its best to defy gravity, and my dull, mud-brown eyes were droopy with tiredness. I poked at my cheeks and scanned myself up and down. I was so weedy. I sighed and began to wash, not half feeling how I looked.

I was quite apprehensive about meeting Dean again, which I knew was silly given that I had seen him *a lot* the day before, as creepily coincidental as it had been. But I was still very much aware of how I had behaved around him, no matter how much I reminded myself not to worry about it. I shook my head violently then, as if to clear my head of any anxiety.

Once all the hard labour was done and I was all set to go, I stared for a long time at my reflection. I had never really studied myself so intently before; it was quite an unnerving feeling, given that I still didn't like what I saw. But I didn't know what else I could do without resorting to drastic plastic surgery measures.

'Well, this is as good as it's gonna get, I suppose,' I said out loud to no-one in particular, bringing my arms abruptly down to my sides in defeat. I then made my way downstairs for breakfast.

The breakfast things were all laid out ready by the time I came down, and as I had half expected, Dean and his mum had already found their seats and were munching away on their toast and cereal. They both looked up at me at the same time when I entered the room.

'Good morning, Laurence, dear. Sleep well?' said Bonnie.

'Very well, thanks.' I nodded. Though feeling Dean's eyes on me, my cheeks began to burn fiercely. I secretly hoped he had noticed my efforts to impress.

'Thanks again for helping me out this morning, mate.' He smiled. 'Really appreciate it.'

'Err, your welcome,' I said quickly, trying to avoid looking directly at him. I found my seat and started on my own food as if I were stocking up for a mission...which I suppose I was, really. In any case, I had to do a lot better than this if I was ever going to impress Dean. He would just think I was a pathetic loser, otherwise.

'So, how long have you guys been running the B&B, then?' Dean asked me, as we made our way down the front garden path twenty minutes later.

'A long time,' I replied shyly. 'About nine or ten years, I think.'

It still didn't feel real, being around Dean. I felt so privileged, but at the same time petrified that I might say something idiotic.

'Well, you guys sure know how to run a business. It's a nice place,' he complimented.

'Thanks. Where are you and your mum from, again?' Though I knew the answer already, I was just trying to keep the conversation flowing without drawing too much attention to my unease.

'We're from Luton originally - just outside of London? So it's a bit weird being all the way out here in the middle of nowhere. I mean, Luton has its countryside, but we were a lot nearer to the town centre there, you know? I'm more used to having things literally on my doorstep. I suppose it's harder getting out and about when you're all the way out here, is it?'

I thought about this. 'Honestly? Yes,' I said, eyes unable to stop themselves from flitting back and forth between Dean and the ground. His gaze always seemed to have a strange affect on me and I was worried he might see this as a sign of weakness.

'Hmm.'

Answer better, Loz!

'I mean, it *is* beautiful out here, but there's absolutely shit all to do,' I blurted, then giggled nervously.

Dean looked a bit shocked, but also impressed by my bold admission and couldn't help but laugh a little, too. I breathed a sigh of relief. It was the truth, though. Suffolk was hardly the most exciting place to live - for people our ages, at least. It was more of a retirement county, or a place to get away to for a quiet weekend break. If you were looking for a good time, you would have to walk several miles to get it! Either that, or wait for the two-hourly bus service to town.

'So, is it just your dad and your...nan who run the place, then?' Dean asked coyly.

'Well, I help out a little, too--'

'Oh, I know! I just...I didn't mean that...Well...' he stuttered, and gestured wildly. He was probably worried he had offended me in some way, but he needn't have been. It was strangely entertaining, though, watching him struggle through *his* words for a change.

'Don't worry, I think I know what you're getting at,' I said gently, finally giving him eye contact. 'I don't have a mum. She, err, died about five years ago from breast cancer.'

'Oh…God, I'm sorry, mate!' And he looked it.

'It's okay, honestly. I suppose it's not all that uncommon these days…Unfortunately.' I smiled up at him weakly. He looked back at me with such sympathy and admiration that it proved a little too much for me, and I had to look away again.

'And, erm, do you, you know,…have a dad at all?' I ventured, trying to turn the attention away from me. It didn't seem all that impertinent a question, really, given that he had just asked about my mum.

'No…Well, yeah, I do, but I don't really see him. He's a dick, anyway. I can't be arsed with him,' he said a little huffily.

'Oh.' I didn't know what else to say to that. It really wasn't my place to pry if he was unwilling to divulge.

'God, this is a bit morbid, isn't it?' He smirked. 'I think we've gone and depressed ourselves.'

I grinned. 'Well, at least all the awkward questions are out of the way, now.'

'Yeah…Oh, hey, is that the bus stop over there?' he said enthusiastically, tilting his head in the direction. 'I spy people!'

Reaching the splintering, wooden-sheltered bus stop, which wasn't all that far down the road from the B&B, we met up with Cyndi Langham, her smarmy-arsed little oik of a brother, Bernard, and Jo Reiner.

Cyndi was a year older than me, most likely in the same sixth form year as Dean - and she was jaw-droppingly gorgeous, it had to be said. She had a near perfect slim-line waist, amazingly wavy, dark hair and glimmering pools of midnight blue for eyes. She was also - though quite unusually given her vanity - one of the loveliest people in my acquaintance. She truly was very sweet.

Her younger brother, Bernard - or Bern - on the other hand, was a freckly, smelly year ten, who, like most of the lower school, thought that in order to make a lasting "cool" impression on the world, much less the school, he had to act like a complete prick 24/7. As brother and sister, the pair couldn't be more dissimilar.

Then there was Jo, a year thirteen who never said or seemed to do much. A pale, gangly girl with long, plaited, light brown hair, I mostly thought she had a lot of the sixth form pride, from which only a few of them suffered. But her kind didn't seem to think it too proper to fraternise with the main-schoolers - aka. The Enemy, aka. me and Bern. So, she tended to keep her snooty self to herself, only ever really acknowledging Cyndi.

'Hey, Loz!' Cyndi called out, waving. Needless to say, the others chose to ignore mine and Dean's oncoming presence.

'Hi, guys!' I called back, if somewhat in vain.

'Hey!' Dean said confidently the closer we got. He certainly wasn't shy! I knew I would have been had I been in his shoes.

'Ooh, hi there!' Cyndi simpered flirtatiously once we were close enough for her to decide that she liked the look of Dean. 'Who's your friend, Loz?'

'This is, erm, Dean, everyone,' I said meekly. 'He's new, and he's living at the B&B with us for a while.'

'Nice to meet you...?'

'Cyndi!' she almost shouted, taking a giant step forward towards him for an even better look, twiddling her beautiful hair banally around her fingers. 'Nice to meet you, too, *Dean*. This is my brother, Bernard, by the way.'

'Bern, *actually*,' Bern snarled, pulling away at the holly bush, which grew through the punctured gaps of the old shelter.

'Hiya,' Dean said to him

Bern didn't bother to reply, though, and Cyndi gave her brother a disparaging look.

'...And that's Jo, over there,' I pointed.

Jo was sitting down on the bench in the shelter, next to Bern, with a face on her like a smacked arse.

'Hi, Jo,' Dean waved.

'Hullo,' she said uninterestedly, not even making the effort to look up at him properly. She was too busy playing with a pebble under her shoe, making an irritating sound on the gravel.

All in all, I was a bit disappointed with Dean's welcome to the village.

'So, Dean, you're in the sixth form, I take it?' Cyndi asked, taking in his profile again.

'That's right.' He nodded.

'Which year?'

'First.'

'Ooh, me too!' she squealed excitedly. She was practically jumping all over him. I liked Cyndi, but she was really starting to bother me all of a sudden. Jo didn't seem to be enjoying the spectacle too much, either, from the look of disgust on her face. 'Maybe you're in one of my classes. Is today your first day, then?'

'Well, no, yesterday was, actually.' He grinned. He obviously didn't seem to mind Cyndi's overindulgence one bit.

'Oh? But I haven't seen you around...'

'It's a big sixth form.' He shrugged. 'I only had a few lessons yesterday, anyway. Then I came straight back here with my mum to settle into the B&B.'

'And why are you at the B&B?' she asked.

'We needed somewhere temporary to stay for a while, since we moved up here pretty hastily.'

'So, where are you from?'

Jeez! What was with all the questions?! She may as well have strapped him to a chair in a poorly lit room and forced the answers out of him with a gun to his head! Why couldn't she just leave him alone?!

'Luton,' he said anyway.

'I thought I could detect a London accent,' she winked, and I grated my teeth. For the first time ever, I really felt as though I could have clunked her! I decided then and there that I did *not* like Cyndi Langham as much as I thought I did anymore!

The bus ride to school was a chore in itself, having to endure tens of annoying kids trying to make themselves known to Dean. He really did seem to captivate people's attention, emitting an irresistible charm.

Since I was the only person he properly knew on the whole bus, he chose to sit by me; this made me feel even more special. I kind of guessed that it would only be a matter of time, though, before he found other more popular friends to sit next to, and then my occasional companionship would no longer be needed. Until then, however, I decided I would make the most of being his temporary lackey.

Looking around the bus, I could see a lot of people thinking the obvious. They were all trying to establish the link between the geek and the potential school heartthrob. But while I was with Dean, no one dared seem brave enough to ask him. This made me smile. They barely knew him and yet, already, he was an untouchable - and I was with him!

At school, we all went our separate ways - the main-schoolers to the horribly aged and grimy-looking main school, and the sixth formers to the newly built and stylishly furnished sixth form block. Dean gave me a manly pat of the shoulder as we leapt off the bus, and nodded his head at me as he walked off with the rest of the sixth form crowd.

I was on cloud nine, as random people came up to me (ones who might not normally even look at me, let alone talk to me, I might add!), demanding to know more about The New Guy. I answered their impatient questions as nonchalantly as possible, with an air of what-makes-you-possibly-think-he'd-be-interested-in-knowing-who-you-are-anyway?, and spent the rest of the morning in a similar mood. This was a far cry from how I had felt the day before, but as I said, I had already established with myself that Dean was merely an idol to me. Maybe we could even be lasting friends. This might not be very likely, but I could always hope.

'You're very *happy* today,' Frankie commented, as she, Zen and I sat down in a shady corner of the playing field at break time.

'Why shouldn't I be?' I asked, cheeks now hurting from smiling so much. 'And anyway, I've always been a happy-go-lucky kind of person. You know that.'

Someone snorted, but I chose to ignore it.

'Well, you're starting to creep me out,' said Zen. 'You're all super smiley and glowy and stuff.'

Frankie laughed and I pouted.

I could have told them what I might have had cause to feel happy about, but they wouldn't have understood. I thought of Dean and another, reflexive smile crept back onto my face. With my newfound no-worries philosophy still intact, I wasn't about to let it bother me, though.

I should probably tell you a little bit about Zen and Frankie, since they already play a pretty big part in my life. They are quite simply my rocks - my best friends. I have known them both for the best part of my life so far and they know me inside and out...well, kind of.

First up, Francesca-Louise Powell - or Frankie, as she prefers. Make the mistake of calling her by her full double-barrelled first name, and you pay with your life! It's just too girly for her liking, she says, and she swears that someday she will have it permanently changed to just *Frankie*. As you can probably guess by that statement, she's a bit of a tomboy in no uncertain way. She has an enviably crazy-wonderful wardrobe - even her uniform is personalised beyond recognition, much to the teachers' and her parents' dismay; and with her great logical outlook on life, Frankie's always the best person to turn to for advice or peace of mind. Oh, and one last thing, she's blatantly hopelessly in love with Zen, but doesn't know it yet.

Zen Stone. Don't ask about the name, his parents are hippies - end of! A little weird and nerdy, with a frightening, Lion King-inspired mane and silly Harry Potter-style glasses, Zen can always manage to bring a smile to your face, whatever your mood - he's a great laugh. But he's also sickeningly head over heels for Frankie, and refuses to admit it. The pair make a ridiculously ideal match, and, had I wanted to give the relationship any fuel, I probably would have said something about it already. But, as it is, I value our little group too much, and should anything happen between the two of them, our threesome would no doubt inadvertently become a twosome.

'I bet I know why you're so happy all of a sudden,' Frankie said.

'Oh, yeah?' I worked hard to make myself seem indifferent.

'I think someone's in luuurve,' she teased, biting the air sexily. I felt Zen twitch beside me. Her statement made me feel all hot and goosepimply, and anxiety shot through me. So much for no-worry philosophies!

'No, that isn't the case at all!' I said a little too defensively.

'Ooh, someone's in denial!' Zen whooped.

'Oh, just get lost!' I snapped, throwing grass blades at them both. They had definitely succeeded in deflating my mood. But they just laughed it off.

'So how are the new guests coming along?' Zen asked, tactfully changing the subject.

'Erm, yeah, they're…great,' I answered, secretly wishing he had changed it to something else.

'Another clueless old couple from London's high-society?' Frankie chipped in.

'Nah, just a mother and son. The son actually goes to the school, he's in the lower sixth form. Name's Dean Mackellar.'

'Never heard of him,' said Zen.

'I think you will do.'

'Why's that?'

'Well…' Oops. 'He just seems like the kind of guy who'll make a lasting impression on the place.'

'Urgh, not one of *those*, is he?' Frankie asked disgustedly. Naturally, by *those* she meant the dickheads who seemed to run the school's corrupt social hierarchy.

'No! God, no! He's a decent guy, I just know he is.'

'Hmm, we'll see about that one.' she said uncertainly.

'From what I can tell, he seems like an all-round nice guy and I really think he'll do well here.'

'*Nice* people never do well in this kind of environment. Not socially, anyway. You should know that, Loz,' Zen said.

I had really had enough of this subject by now.

At that moment, however, I heard footsteps, giggling and chatter closing in on us. And just as I turned round to see which possible annoying toss-pots were coming over to make their sentiments about us known in order to look big in front of their underachieving, chavvy posse, I was surprised to see Dean. He was walking with Cyndi Langham and a few others, not all of whom I recognised - all sixth formers, though. I felt a sudden, though not altogether alien, pang in the pit of my stomach. I was all nerves again and didn't know what to do with myself. The group partially separated while Dean came over to talk to us, Cyndi in tow. Apparently, she was his extended shadow, now.

'Hey, guys!' they called in unison. *Urgh*!

'Hey,' I said quietly, half-smiling. Zen and Frankie looked ready to pounce on them with a few choice words if they dared to challenge us. They clearly had no idea who they were.

'Guys, this is Dean...and Cyndi from my village, remember?' I said, quickly turning back round to reassure them.

They understood instantly and relaxed a little, but I could tell by their body language that they still weren't entirely comfortable with this strange company.

Once they reached us, Dean bent down to our level and got up close to me. My heart raced. He was almost too close.

'A-and Dean,...Cyndi, these are my mates, Zen and Frankie.'

The group exchanged greetings.

'We were just talking about you,' Zen said unwittingly. I could have kicked him!

'Oh? About what?' Dean asked me curiously.

'Err,' I stuttered, 'just letting them know that you're one of our new tenants, that's all...'

Everyone was looking at me, and I did what I do best and coloured.

'Ah, right,' he said almost dismissively before moving off topic. 'Anyway, just thought I'd let you know...I won't be coming back on the bus tonight. The guys, here, have offered to chaperon me around Bury town centre. Nice, huh?'

'Oh,...yeah...nice. Well, sure, don't worry about it. I'll let your mum know, if that's what you mean,' I said weakly. He was making me feel all weird again, with him being so near to me. He was maddeningly handsome up close and he had to go now!

The forced eye contact was killing me, too, and the fact that the smell of him was so immensely pleasing didn't help matters much. I had never had the opportunity to appreciate his scent before - a blend of individual musk and a lightly sweetened aftershave. I sighed inwardly. It was nice, and it made me feel prickly all over.

'Yeah, cool, thanks. I'll see you in a bit, then?' he said as he got up to go. 'Bye, guys.' He nodded.

'Seeya,' I squeaked.

He grinned back at me, then went back to the rest of his group with Cyndi practically draped all over him. That especially burned me up - the flirt!

'Bye, Loz, babe,' she hollered back. I just wanted to chase after her and trip her up!

I then mentally slapped myself for the thought. What was coming over me? I had never disliked Cyndi before - certainly not to this degree! She was the school's answer to female perfection and, typically, I should have found her groin-achingly attractive. At any rate, it wasn't as if she had done or said anything in particular to upset me recently.

Except that she had. She was getting cosy with Dean and that was enough.

Realisation seeped in fast, and I excused myself from Zen and Frankie's side to go to the loo before they had a chance to notice or say anything about my flustered behaviour.

I ran straight to the nearest toilets - in the Science block - and locked myself in a cubicle. Fortunately, no-one was around to hear my hushed sobs, as I slowly came to the conclusion that I did indeed have a crush on Dean - a *gay* crush, no less!

It was scarily obvious now that I thought about it. I was beginning to feel anxious and it was getting harder to breathe. Every pulsating urge I had felt for him each time he was around; being unable to keep eye contact for fear of blushing; and the sheer fact that I was now hugely jealous of Cyndi's budding relationship with him. It all made sense, but it was also all far too irrational. I had known Dean little more than a day, and yet, already, he had managed to turn my entire world upside down. I had never met or seen anyone quite like him before, and I was no longer sure of myself as I once thought I was.

But okay, so maybe I had a *Dean* thing, but then who wouldn't? He was an Adonis with a genuinely sweet temperament to match - you don't often find that. It didn't necessarily mean I had a *guy* thing. And besides, crushes pass. From what I heard, they come and go like fashion trends. I just had to do my best to ride this one out, and hope that maybe someday soon all these feelings would simply be brushed under the rug and left forgotten. I felt myself calm down considerably, and I wiped my cheeks dry.

Just then, the bell rang, signalling the start of class, again. P.E. - great! I could sense the cruel irony there, and so I unwillingly gathered myself together and went out to face the world. Only this time, I felt somewhat vulnerable; as though I had been invisibly, but permanently, branded as *different*; as though people would instantly suss me out and that I would be outcast forever.

'Oh, Dean! Why can't you just go back to where you came from?! It's all your bloody fault!'

CHAPTER 4.

I made my way over to the gym block and into the changing rooms. Mr Loos, a lanky, no-nonsense Australian, was signing people in on the register as they entered the building.

'I hope you continue to have your kit with you this year, Mr Price,' Mr Loos said, pointing his pen at the dangling plastic bag at my side as I slid past him.

I just rolled my eyes away from him and muttered, 'Yes, sir.'

I hated P.E. Not necessarily just because I disliked the majority of sports that we played, but mostly because it was such a cliquey subject. It was practically the only one where the rowdier lads took themselves seriously in, but to the extent that they would exclude or humiliate anyone who wasn't up to scratch on their footy skills. It was much easier to accidentally on purpose forget to bring in your kit each week. Then again, you did have to hope that the lost property bin would be conveniently empty of "spare" P.E. clothes that day.

The changing room benches were almost full, but I managed to squeeze onto an end space. I could hear loutish whooping and messing around behind me. I knew what was coming.

'Alright, Pricey?' Jammy roared, finally noticing me.

Oh, joy! Jammy - James Jobson - was the year group arsehole. He was as bad as they came. He was constantly in trouble with teachers, never did any work, and was an all-round bully. And I was his favourite target!

Every time he even caught a whiff of me, he just couldn't resist saying something incredibly spiteful and unnecessary just to big himself up in front of his mates. By the end of last year, though, I had got pretty good at avoiding him. Unless I happened to share a class with him, that is. Otherwise, I could pretty much work out his timetable, and so tended to know where he would be at what time. Outside the classroom, as well, I was only ever occasionally unfortunate enough to bump into him. I would need to get a head start this term, if I wanted another relatively Jammy-free year.

'You actually gonna play something this year, Pricey?' Jammy sneered. His half naked, hyena-like friends heckled away behind him while they changed.

'Dunno. Are you actually gonna do any work this year, Jammy?' I replied sarcastically, giving him an I'm-not-really-in-the-mood-for-this-shit kind of look. Not that I ever was, but more so not today than any other.

'Ooh! Harsh, man!' his friends jeered and clapped. Spectators stifled their laughter and applause, lest the bullying turned onto them instead.

He snickered. 'Well, I dunno, mate. You gonna suck on the teachers' knobs just so you can be their pet again this year?'

This time, the whole changing room couldn't contain itself, and I went crimson with a mixture of rage and embarrassment.

'I mean, you gotta give someone else a chance,' he continued. 'Know what I mean, mate?'

I glared at him, but he just mocked away, making inappropriate sucking gestures. If he was trying to make me feel small and stupid, he was going the right way about it - he was a gold medallist at that! Whenever he started on me I could always come up with at least one good one-line comeback, but when he carried on like that I just lost the will to fight it. It wouldn't be worth it in the end, and I certainly didn't fancy having a broken face any time soon. When faced with a burly, ugly half-wit with only brute strength and cockiness to recommend him, resistance was almost futile

Fortunately, Mr Loos came in in time before things could get any worse, and started telling us all about how the year's sports timetable would pan out. For the time being it was football and rugby, which was just great for me because of course I absolutely loved having virtually frost bitten limbs week after week throughout the winter months! Meanwhile, however, my legs would just have to make the most of the final weeks of nice weather we were being blessed with.

Just then, two lads walked in from the P.E. staff room, dressed in tracksuits. My stomach almost jumped right up out of my mouth.

'Right, guys. I'd like to introduce you all to your new sixth form sports reps for the year: Dean Mackellar and Randal Nielson,' Mr Loos said.

It would be Dean, wouldn't it! I hadn't anticipated this, but it was typical of my luck. Why did it seem like I couldn't get away from him? I suppose, though, that there always was a slight possibility it would be him. It was fairly obvious from his athletic physique that he enjoyed his exercise.

Sports reps were sixth form P.E. students who spent the majority of their lessons helping the teachers teach us. They all specialised in certain areas of sport for their exams and coursework, and took the opportunity to help us as an excuse for extra credit for university applications as well as for revision purposes. Of course, being that they probably knew half the class from around the school and were friends with them already, it was difficult for them not to play favourites. The less keen members of the class were, therefore, still ignored. But if they were anything like me, they would only have been grateful.

Now, though, I was beginning to feel unusually driven, and it wasn't hard to think why. The urge to impress Dean had come back. I just had to prove I wasn't a complete waste of space, and that I could be as worthy of his esteem as the rest of the thick-as-shit jocks in the class. I knew I would never be able to reach their standard of sporting skill, but I could at least try, for him.

I scolded myself again for my thoughts, but then sighed in defeat as I glanced over at him, who, once he saw me, gave me a little warm smile in recognition. As always, something inside me jump-started and I turned away, all flustered.

Once the pep talk was over and done with, we were then sorted into our groups. Half and half. One half was to do football, the other to do rugby, and then each week we would alternate. This week was football for me and, unfortunately, so was it for Jammy & Co.

Since P.E. was not a graded subject and only a legal requirement for under-sixteens in fulltime education as part of a weekly health and fitness programme enforced by the government, I never really took time to notice what the proper rules for any of the sports were. I had a vague inclination as to how they were played, of course, but that had always been more than enough for me. I would have to start paying attention, now, I guess.

Next, we were assigned our sports rep. Naturally, Dean was ours. I didn't know whether to be glad or worried. Part of me wanted to show off to him, but then something else inside me didn't want me to make a fool out of myself, as I knew showing off would only highlight all the more how spectacularly crap I was at sports.

Out on the playing field, Dean sprinted over to us. He introduced himself informally to the guys and chatted about some game strategies - all of which meant absolutely nothing to me. However, there was instant respect among the rest of the group for him. This surprised me hugely, especially given that he was dealing with some of the roughest lads in the whole of East Anglia! But then, he had a confident, charismatic air about him, which was very easy to be seduced by. There was only a year's age gap between us, but already the guys treated him as a form of authority figure. I couldn't help but feel proud of him for managing that. Mr Loos looked happy enough, too, with Dean's progress, as he drifted between the groups, gradually spending more and more time helping out Randal with the rugby lads than with us.

We did a little warm up jog before getting started, and then the teams were picked, and Dean did the picking. He obviously didn't have a clue as to how much Jammy and I detested one another, because I was, once again, lumbered with him and the rest of his slack-jawed crew.

Our team got off to a flying start, in spite of my participation. And in all fairness, I did try my best to involve myself; even attempting to look as though I actually knew what was going on - not an easy task, I can tell you!

As far as I was concerned, football was a bit of a yoyo game. Back and forth with the ball, a kick here, a header there, and then... GOAL!, apparently. Pretty monotonous and pointless, but simple enough, I guess. It really was far too competitive for what it was, though.

However, just to add further injustice to my situation, regardless of whether we were any good or not, Dean made sure that everyone had a turn in goal. All the lads' lads took to this duty with great gusto. I mean, this is their livelihood we are talking about - when they are not busy bunking off lessons, of course.

When it came to my turn, Jammy and his mates were in uproar. Being on their team, they knew as well as I did that I was rubbish, but what they didn't know was that this time I was going to try to deliberately not be. I had to; my reputation as an acquaintance of Dean's was at stake, here!

I rushed over to take Jammy's place, who I could tell was not too happy about relinquishing his current position as goalie to a far inferior candidate; to someone who barely looked strong enough to withstand the wind, let alone take a ball to the head.

'You better fucking try, Pricey!' he scowled, giving me a rough shove, then jogged past me to get back into the game. I just pulled a face after him.

The good thing about being in goal - or more precisely, the only good thing about being in goal - was that, though the job was important - ensuring the team's security within the game by protecting the weak spot - most of the time when the ball was anywhere else but within the goal posts, you could make the most of not getting too involved. You could even relax a little, without feeling forced to aimlessly chase after a cheap, half-deflated rubber ball.

I didn't get a chance to relax for long, however, before the conflicting stampede made its way over to me. My body shook with fear as it always did whenever I was goalkeeper, praying that my team would fend off the opposition so as to save myself from the inevitable shame of failing to defend.

'Heads up, queer boy!' a voice I didn't recognised shouted, as the ball was booted my way.

Queer boy?

'Wha--?' was all I could muster before the ball ricocheted off my nose, the sheer force of it causing me to fall flat onto my back onto the dusty, worn-away ground.

I had successfully defended the home goal, but at a price. My nose was now flooding blood, streaking down the front of my P.E. top. The pain was immense, as I tried, rather unsuccessfully, to fight back the tears. I couldn't be seen as a weakling, especially not in front of Dean.

The whistle sounded, and Mr Loos, Dean and both teams came rushing over to me.

Well, so much for sportsmanship! Not one of my team members dared come close enough to help me out. They just stood there, gawping and tittering at the humorousness of it all, occasionally making discomforted noises. Dean and Mr Loos, on the other hand, helped me to my feet, and Mr Loos then suggested that Dean escort me to the sick bay straightaway. He didn't hesitate, and before I knew it, I was whisked off the pitch and taken indoors to be cleaned up.

'Thanks for your help,' I said to Dean in a muffled voice from under my tissue, which was held firmly on my throbbing nose to soak up any excess blood. We were both sitting outside the nurse's office, waiting for me to get the all-clear to go back to class. I felt so undignified in front of Dean like this. I hadn't seen myself, but I was sure looked a right state, especially with my once bleached-white polo shirt now dyed scarlet.

Luckily for me, though, the only damage done was a burst blood vessel and a bruise the size of Britain across the middle of my face for all my trouble - no broken bones just yet. I wasn't exactly sure how qualified the sick bay nurse was at giving out such diagnoses, but I chose to trust her judgement. I mean, my nose did still feel like it was in its usual place, and I wasn't bleeding as much anymore.

'No worries, mate,' Dean said. 'It's just the luck of the game sometimes, I guess.'

I half-choked.

'You call this luck?' My voice must have sounded funny with tissue up my nostrils, as I could see him trying to suppress a giggle.

'...You know what I mean.'

I harrumphed. 'Well, I suppose it doesn't really matter much, does it? I know I'm crap and the others know it, too--'

'I do know it was on purpose, Loz,' he interjected. 'And don't worry, I'll be giving the little shit who did it a thing or two to think about later!'

'Oh, no, you really don't have to! This kinda thing is pretty

routine for me…Well, not so much bloodied noses, but you know…'
I shrugged.

'Yeah, I know.' He smiled understandingly. 'Just leave it to me, though, okay?'

'Dean, I appreciate it, but…'

He put his finger to his lips as if to silence me, and gave me a mischievous wink. I blushed fiercely.

I was in awe of his apparent protectiveness of me, and as I scanned his beautifully symmetrical features, I didn't know what else to say. He just looked back at me, empathy written all over him. When the awkward silence finally dawned on me, I pretended to be all hot and bothered.

Why did he want to look out for me? Nobody else did. Well, except Zen and Frankie, but then they were my best friends and would always defend me to the ground. But Dean was virtually a stranger, and he was only living with me for the time being. Other than that, we had no ties. Why did he care so much?

'Anyway,' he continued, 'I have strong morals, and just because you're strong it doesn't give you the right to pick on those weaker than yourself.'

I was a little stung by his tactlessness. He was just acting charitable, and saw me little more than a defenceless coward.

The sick bay nurse came out then, mercifully butting in, and after double checking that my nose was indeed not broken, she was happy enough to let me go.

'Bollocks! I've really gotta run, dude,' Dean said, rising quickly to his feet and looking at the little clock on his mobile. 'I was supposed to be in Maths ten minutes ago!'

'Oh. Well, sure, if you've got to go…I'm mean, I've got a French test to get to, anyway…Once changed, of course.' I giggled nervously, looking down at my blood-sodden shirt.

He smiled again. 'Well, listen, mind the nose,' he motioned to my swelling, 'and I'll catch you later tonight.'

'Yeah, thanks. Oh, and have fun in town. I'm sure your friends will show you a good time.'

He gave me a corny thumbs up, then sprinted off down the corridor to his lesson. My eyes wandered after him.

So he did do Maths after all. For some reason it didn't seem so awful a subject anymore.

Later, at home time, I noticed a group of lads from my P.E. class walking by, on their way to the buses. At the sight of me, however, one of the lads - whose right cheek was noticeably more rouged than the left - looked panicked and pulled his mates away in the opposite direction, encouraging them to move on as quickly as possible. From his reaction, I construed it to mean two things: the first being that my, now mercilessly distended, nose was so grotesque, or second, that Dean had kept his word and set him straight. I went with the latter, grinning broadly to myself. Dean had my back.

That evening, I was purposefully being antisocial and barricaded myself in my room. My own company was all I needed. There wasn't much left to analyse in my head, now, as I pretty much knew how I felt about Dean. He had come into my life and I wasn't the same anymore - certainly not the same person I was yesterday morning. An unwelcome, though ever curious, change had come about me. And that evening, as I sat up in my bedroom perched on the low windowsill, attempting to decipher *Twelfth Night* for English Lit., all I could think of doing was looking out for a car that might be bringing Dean back home.

CHAPTER 5.

The next day, on our way to the bus stop, Dean and I chatted and joked. Conversation flow was a lot easier between us today. Maintained eye contact was becoming more bearable, too...to a degree, as I was trying harder to create a better impression of myself. However, yesterday's P.E. palaver, where I had all but lost all dignity I had, had left me still a tiny bit shy of him.

Pointing out that the inflammation around my nose had marginally reduced since, I thanked him for whatever it was he had said or done to the little football punk in my defence.

I even found out a little bit more about Dean - the minor details of his life were no longer such a mystery. I found myself completely fascinated by the things he said. Even the seemingly trivial facts, like what school he went to before (Worley High School), what he studied in sixth form now (P.E. - duh, Maths - duh, and Physics - not all that surprising, I guess), and whether or not he was learning to drive yet (No, as his seventeenth birthday wasn't for another month), still left me hungry for more.

I was also eager to know what he thought about town. I didn't get a chance to ask the night before, since he had got home later than I was physically capable of keeping my eyes open for.

'Mum gave me such a bollocking when I got in, you know,' he boasted.

'I bet! I was wondering when you'd show up. Out late on a school night!'

'Aw, worried, were you?' he teased.

'Course not!' Though I turned away quickly before I could blush, because I actually had been a little. 'I'm sure Cyndi took good care of you.'

'Yeah, they're all safe.'

'Who were the others you went with, then? Other than Cyndi,' I asked.

'Just a couple of guys - a few off of my courses: Randal Nielson and Harry Fitzgibbons. And that Jobson guy from your year,' he said.

I came to a halt.

'What's wrong?'

'Jobson? You mean, *Jammy* Jobson, right?'

'Sure. That, or James.' He shrugged. 'What's wrong?'

'Let's just say Jammy and I don't exactly see eye to eye, that's all.' I said stiffly, as I walked on a bit past him.

'Why's that?' he persisted.

'I dunno. Because he's a twat, probably,' I muttered.

'Well, he was alright with me.'

'Well, he would be, because you're a lot cooler than I am,' I explained.

Dean just laughed and I went red again.

'You think I'm "cool"?' He smiled quizzically.

'Well….I, err…'

'I've never been called "cool" before. That's cute, that is,' he chuckled.

'Shut-up!' I smirked, while trying to hide my humiliation.

We walked on. A painfully awkward pause followed.

'So what did you get up to in town, then?' I asked almost shrilly, attempting to move things on.

He kicked at the gravel beneath his feet as he strolled. 'Nothing much, really. We chilled in the park for a bit, had a few, went to Mackie-Dee's, and just generally hung around.'

'Oh?' I said. 'A few…?'

'Drinks, of course!' he laughed in disbelief of my apparent ignorance.

'Oh, I know, but I thought you were still, you know, *underage.*'

'I am, but if you can get away with it…'

'…Ah, okay.' I had so much to learn.

'You'll have to come out with us next time,' he said easily, causing me to almost stop dead in my tracks again. Did he just say what I thought he said?

'You want *me* to come out with *you*…next time?' I spluttered.

'Sure, why not?'

This *was* an honour! Honestly, anyone would have thought I had been granted a knighthood by the Queen! Then again, not even that, I'm sure, would have been able to equal how I felt at this moment in time. Was Dean finally recognising my attributes as a potential friend?

And then I thought of Jammy.

'Oh, I…just, I dunno.'

'Look, if you're worried about James, you don't have to be. He's a nice enough guy, really. You probably just got off on the wrong foot,' he assured.

I grumbled. 'I seriously doubt it's that.'

'I'm just saying…'

I thought it over quickly. The most good-looking and newly most popular guy around was asking me to socialise with him, and all I would have to do was put up with Jammy The Arsehole for a couple of hours. And anyway, I was he wouldn't dare say too much to me in front of Dean and the others…or would he?

'Okay, sure,' I finally agreed, throwing caution to the wind. I was starting to really look forward to this again.

'Hi, guys!' Cyndi called out from inside the beckoning bus shelter.

My mood soured instantly. If it wasn't Jammy I would have to contend with, it would definitely be *her*!

CHAPTER 6.

'So, what are your plans this weekend?' Frankie asked as we walked down the corridor to our last lesson of the day.

It was Friday afternoon, and tomorrow was going to be the day that I was going to spend with Dean and his new friends. Of course, I hadn't told Zen and Frankie about it - they wouldn't understand. They would see me as a traitor to everything we stood for. They would think I was trying to muscle in on the "It" crowd, to gain popularity points. So I lied, and told them I was just going to be spending some time helping my dad clean the house and doing coursework. What they didn't know wouldn't hurt them, I reasoned.

'Alright. But give us a ring. Zen will be round mine on Sunday if you want to join us. We'll just be chillin' out on the village green,' she said, as we entered Mr Crawley's Maths classroom.

I said I would think about it.

'Let's go out tonight!' Dean announced that same evening, standing in my bedroom doorway. He looked fresh-faced and dashing in a tight-ish-fitted, black, long-sleeved shirt, rolled up at the arms and finished off with expensive-looking jeans and brown slip-ons. I was a little unprepared for all this, to say the least, so my heart could be forgiven for doing little flips at the sight of him.

'What? Tonight? But, but...' I sputtered.

'Yeah, I know we're out tomorrow, but to hell with it! I'm bored as fuck here,' he whined, frustrated.

'Erm, okay, but what will there be for us to do? The shops will be shut by now,' I said naively.

He just laughed at me. 'Err, go clubbing, of course! Duh!'

'But…' I panicked a little. I had never been clubbing before, not least because I wasn't old enough!

'Come on! There's this wicked bar I went to last week with the guys. We had a right laugh, and there's loads of eye candy!' Dean said excitedly, making my heart drop several feet as I realised what his real intention in going out was - to hook up.

As much as I denied it, I wasn't interested in "eye candy." I was interested in *him*. Still, for the sake of being with him, I was easily persuaded to go along. It would be an experience, at least. And who knew? Maybe a girl *would* catch my eye.

'How will I even get into places? There's no-way I could pass for 18!' I complained.

He tapped his nose slyly. 'Leave that one to me.'

Of all the people he could have chosen to go out with I couldn't understand why he had chosen me, but I wasn't going to argue that point with him. Dean was taking me out!…Even if it was in possible pursuit of a girlfriend.

'Aren't we going with anyone else, then?' I enquired, while rummaging through my drawers for something special to wear.

'Nah, too much hassle. We're seeing the guys tomorrow. But you never know, we might meet them out later, too.

'Anyway, I've lived with you for almost two weeks, now, and we still haven't done anything together as just us two housemates yet, have we?'

'Alright.' I beamed, now agreeing whole-heartedly to the idea. Inwardly, I was jumping for joy; at least we would be bonding. Then I stopped what I was doing, taking in for a second time what Dean was wearing. 'How did you know I'd eventually agree to this?' I asked, one eyebrow raised.

He just smiled shrewdly, then turned and left, leaving me to it.

In the end, I decided on one of my seldom worn tops - my green V-neck, and my least scruffy pair of jeans. I didn't have many nice shoes, so had to settle for my school shoes. I then scrutinised myself in the mirror, which was becoming a habitual routine for me these days, and again decided I would have to make do with what I saw. At least my nose swelling was less noticeable, now.

'Very smart,' Dean approved, standing in the hallway waiting, as I made my way downstairs.

Though I still didn't think it was wholly deserved, his appreciation sent an unexplained thrill through me. I then realised that that was what I must have been subconsciously aiming for.

We told the parents we were going into town to watch a film, and that then we would maybe go round one of Dean's mates' houses for a bit. And like all oblivious parents believing their children to be the exception to the teen rebellion rule, they lapped it up.

We took the 337 bus at 7:20pm to the town centre and headed straight for the pubs for a few drinks before the nightlife really got started.

Dean went over to the bars with such confidence and ease that even I half believed that he wasn't underage. He was unbelievable, and he hardly ever got ID'd. I mostly stayed out of sight - tucked away safely in the corner, racking up the balls on the snooker table, or else I hid in the toilets while he did his thing. Then we just chatted and laughed away the evening, played on the slot machines and spent our winnings on the next round. It was a lot of fun, and as the night wore on, I became steadily more and more drunk. Who would have thought a few bottles of Smirnoff Ice (as I didn't like beer, much to Dean's disapproval) could get you off your face! It wasn't a lot, to be honest, but then I had still never drunk as much in any one sitting before. I didn't initially like the alcohol; I wasn't much accustomed to the taste. But as the rounds kept on coming, the more I found I enjoyed my tipple.

'*Psst*, Loz! Check them out...over there!' Dean whispered loudly across the table to me.

It was now 10:00pm and we were in The Vines - a trendy joint - our fourth stop on our pub crawl, on our fifth round of drinks, and we were clearly suffering. The place was packed, and we were happy in our drunken stupor in a dark corner behind the crowds - out of eyeshot of suspecting bar staff - and busy checking out the "talent."

'Eh...where?' I leaned across to see, feigning interest.

'That 'un over there.' He pointed a wobbly finger over towards a pair of female figures standing in front of the cigarette machine by the door.

'Oh...Bleurgh! You mean the one who looks a bit lesbian-y?'

He laughed heartily.

'Pfff, nah! Her mate, the blonde - the one with the melons. The lesbian's got rubbish tits, anyway,' he slurred.

I decided to take his word for it. I squinted at the blonde. 'Ah, *her*. Yeah, she's alright, I s'pose,' I sighed, collapsing back into my seat. To her credit, and to my sudden annoyance, she *was* actually quite attractive.

Dean then turned to me. 'So, anyway, Mr Price...'

'Hmm?'

'What kinda girls do you, you know, *go for*?'

I pondered this. 'Erm, I've never really thought 'bout it much.' I really hadn't.

'Eh? Really? Come on, there's gotta be *some* girl at school you've got your eye on.'

'Nope,' I said too quickly.

He chortled, 'Sure you ain't gay?'

I choked a little on my drink and sobered up almost instantly. Thankfully, before I could defend myself, he got up and said, 'I'm gonna go get us some more drinks. Same again, mate?'

'Y-yeah, please.' I stammered in relief, and watched him stumble a little way over to the bar. That was far too close for comfort! I was feeling incredibly uneasy, now.

Minutes later, he was back again with a pint of Carling for himself and a vodka and lemonade for me. I realised early on that I needed to upgrade from alco-pops to something a little stronger if I ever wanted to battle my nerves of getting caught out. The more confident I came across to bouncers, the better.

'I still dunno how you don't like beers - they're gorgeous!' Dean slurped clumsily on his fresh glass as he sat down.

'I don't know how you *can*! Tastes like liquidised bread,' I argued, scrunching up my face. He couldn't seem to help but laugh at me again. 'Besides, drinking vodka mixers is sort of like drinking pop - they're easy.'

He just rolled his eyes in defeat. 'Right...Well, we'll finish this round off and then it's straight to a club, okay? Wanna try that one by the chippy?'

'You mean Club Toulouse?'

'That's the one! My mate, Harry, his brother's a bouncer there.

He's well safe. If he's working tonight he'll let us in - no problem,' he said, resuming looking back at the blonde with her ambiguous-looking friend.

Whatever he was doing with those magical eyes of his obviously worked a treat, because it wasn't long before Blondie couldn't resist looking over in our direction, either. Eventually, she turned to her friend as if persuading her to come over with her to say 'hi.' The friend didn't seem all that impressed at first, but when she saw where Melon-ie was looking, her face lit up as well.

'Safe! Got'em to come over. Right, dibs on the blonde, yeah?' Dean said quietly, rubbing his hands together like a greedy businessman. He was so hopelessly straight. A part of me pined for him right there and then; he was just so perfect – practically unobtainable. I defied anyone to not to want him. All I could think was how much I wished I was in that lucky bitch's shoes right now, to be allowed to like him and be liked by him in that way in return. She should feel lucky enough to even be able to breathe the same air as him, let alone walk up to him!

A not altogether uncommon emotion was stirring, just like it had done before with Cyndi Langham. I was green with envy, and the darker side of me wanted to punch this imposing bimbo right in the chesticles and poke her eyes out with my drink's straw. I didn't need to get to know her to know I hated her already!

'Hi,' she said sweetly, once she and her friend had sauntered their way over to our little table.

Tramp! growled a sinister-sounding voice from deep within the depths of my mind.

'Hey.' Dean nodded, sounding as chilled out as possible.

'Saw you checkin' us out over there.'

Urgh! it went again

'Oh yeah?'

'Yeah,' she said flirtatiously

Slapper!

'I'm Donna, by the way. And this is my mate, Holly.'

Bugger off!

'Nice to meet you, ladies. I'm Dean, and this is *my* mate, Loz.'

'Nice to meet you,' the girl presumed to be Donna said, leering at me. 'I think Holl well fancies *you*, babe.'

Holly went crimson, and gave Donna a quick elbow in the ribs while muttering something sharply in her ear.

Great. I had a repressed lesbian admirer.

'He's all yours,' Dean said to Holly, giving me a nudge under the table.

I just wanted to run away.

Meanwhile, the girls took to their seats either side of us - Holly next to me, of course.

'So how old are you guys, anyway?' Donna chirped, running her finger around the rim of her drink's glass seductively.

'Both eighteen,' Dean answered coolly

'Cool.'

I presumed her answer meant that either they were, too, or that they were just glad to know that we were at least old enough to be drinking in a bar. At any rate, I knew asking a strange lady her age was a bit of a social taboo, but to hell with it! I didn't exactly want them around any longer.

'And you guys? How old are you?' I asked, confidently. I must still have been more drunk than I thought. Dean shot me a glance.

The girls didn't seem too put out, though, and were happy enough to tell us that they were both twenty - shit! This felt so wrong on so many levels. I was barely legal, and I wanted out!

'You know, you guys still look pretty young for eighteen. You hardly look old enough to shave. Sure you ain't fibbin'?' Donna ventured, biting lightly on her bottom lip.

'Would have been thrown out by now, wouldn't we?' Dean said just as easily.

'Eh, s'pose so.'

'Fancy another round?' he asked everyone.

So much for heading straight to the club!

'Sure, I'll come with you,' Donna said, getting up.

Dean gave me a cheeky wink as he turned to the bar, arm in arm with her, leaving me alone with the ever silent Holly.

I turned to her and made an attempt at a smile. She looked about as comfortable as I did.

'So, erm, do you come here much?' she asked shyly.

At least it could speak.

'Err, no. First time, actually. I don't really get to go out much,' I replied quickly.

'Oh?'

'Yeah. Busy, see.'

'Oh.'

And that was the extent of our conversation. I was sorry to disappoint her, but I couldn't have been more uninterested.

In all fairness, I suppose the girl wasn't that bad looking. Maybe a little plain, but she did have a nice, trim body working in her favour, even if, as Dean had correctly observed, she wasn't exactly blessed in the cleavage department. Her hair was the only really offending part about her, making her look as though she had been attacked by a lunatic with a set of secateurs.

Luckily, to put us out of our misery just in time before I contemplated drowning myself in my dregs, Dean and Donna came waddling back over with a tray of shots.

'Sambucas all round!' Donna trilled.

'On me, of course - enjoy!' Dean said. Everyone but me took their glass and downed it in one gulp, wincing and retching over the aftertaste. I was biding my time with mine. I had never had a shot before, and from the looks on their faces, it didn't look as though it tasted very nice.

'Down it, boy, c'mon!' Donna cajoled.

'Erm, in a minute, maybe.'

'C'mon, chug!'

I stared at the little glass.

'Chug! Chug! Chug!' all three of them chanted until I finally gave in. In one swift motion, I downed the whole thing, though not without almost throwing it back up again over Holly. It was disgusting - like black liquorish juice with a deadly kick. I certainly didn't want another one of those anytime soon! The others just fell about laughing at my comical expressions.

'Right, then. Who's up for Toulouse?' Dean shouted, shooting right up out of his seat again. The way he said it made it sound as if he meant to invite Bimborella and the hairdresser's worst nightmare to join us, too!

'Ooh, I do!' Donna bounced about stupidly.

I wanted to slap her. The girl's methods of flirtation were idiotic at best.

Holly just shuffled uncomfortably in her seat next to me. I could see that she had had enough of mine and Dean's company, now, after finally realising that I couldn't be bothered with her.

'Right, powder room first!' Donna said, grabbing her friend by the arm and literally dragging her. Holly couldn't have looked gladder to get away, if only for a little bit.

'You're inviting *them*, too?' I hissed, reaching up to Dean's height.

'Sure, why not? They're cool, right?' he yawned, leaning against the wall.

'They're a bit annoying, actually.' I muttered.

'Wha--?' he said with an edge of irritation.

'Nothing.'

Club Toulouse was rammed - as expected for a Friday night - and as Dean had predicted, his mate Harry's brother, Freddie, was doorman. With a knowing wink, he let us right in - Donna and Dean walking together, holding each other up, and me and Holly keeping close to either side of them.

Once inside, however, we lost Holly almost instantly, as she shot off towards a small group of girls waiting around one of the already crowded bars. Either they were friends of hers or she was just so desperate to get away from us that she had managed to forge new friendships in the middle of the club. Though relieved to, at last, be rid of her, I hoped for her sake it was the first.

Donna hadn't even noticed that Holly had gone, or so it seemed. She was too busy gyrating up and down Dean in the middle of the dance floor to care. I watched on, appalled, from afar, sensibly waiting in line at the opposite bar to where Holly and her "other" friends were, who weren't trying very hard to make it look as if they weren't talking about me.

I was officially miserable, and I only had a tenner left of my allowance on me. But to hell with it, I decided. If I was going to survive the night, I needed to be pissed out of my mind! I was already feeling a slight buzz, though arguably more so after the foul-tasting shot than anything else I had had that night. But it was my ferocious jealousy that was overpowering everything else, keeping me from truly having a good time. I needed to drink so much past that emotion that I wouldn't even be able to understand the meaning of the word, let alone feel it.

I no longer felt frightened about being sussed out at the bar, seeing as if I was really going to be kicked out for being underage, they would have done it at the door already. I then, begrudgingly, braced myself for a round of three Sambuca shots - as they were the only brand I knew of - and a bottle of WKD to help wash things down.

The next thing I remember was being on the dance floor. Donna and Dean were nowhere in sight, and I appeared to be having a brilliant time, dancing about, looking like God-only-knows-what, with an athletic broad moving energetically about me in a hideous, orange dress that felt like crepe paper. That memory went on for a while, but whatever else followed remained a blur.

⁊

It was 1.30am in Club Toulouse and Dean was bored. He stood to the side with half a pint in his hands, grimacing at the sight in front of him. Donna was drunk, and she was making ill use of the dancing pole she spun around on the little platform in the middle of the dance floor. He was just glad she was out of the way.

He had fast grown tired of her and really didn't know why he had bothered with her in the first place. He guessed it had something to do with wanting to live up to Loz's high expectation of him, to be the guy he thought Loz thought he was - just for a laugh, at least. He had quite enjoyed playing up to this supposed unattainable role model. It was kind of fun, and he had, admittedly, unfairly milked it for a while. But he was fed up now, no longer enjoying being the kind of promiscuous person he had played out to be. And anyway, Donna was far from his usual type.

There were five other random girls - clad in stilettos and skimpy tops and oversized belts - fighting their way around the tiny podium, vying for extra space to show off their nonexistent skills. It was quite funny to watch, actually, Dean thought. Especially with the equally intoxicated guys encircling them hungrily, like a group of horny apes, whooping and reaching out for them, unashamedly pulling at their skirts for more. Even the DJ frequently commented on how "great" they looked, bribing them all with a free bottle of champagne for whoever pole-danced the best. An unofficial competition was hence started. Dean just rolled his eyes heavenwards. He was losing his buzz. The music wasn't as good as promised, and the scene really wasn't his.

He was only really here for Loz's sake - his first night to a club, after all. It was always best to start somewhere small and then work your way up, as he himself had learnt. The more club savvy you were while underage, the more successful you would hopefully be at worming your way into more prestigious joints. There was one club in particular in Ipswich that was supposedly infamous here in the east. It was called Flame, and Dean was determined to get Loz in there at some point. It was ten times better than this poor excuse for a shack, not so cleverly disguised as a nightclub in the middle of nowhere.

Yes, Flame would be perfect - a far better scene. His kind of scene. *Their* kind of scene. It would show Loz once and for all, would make him understand what it was he was missing. Dean just wanted to break him free of his constraints, show him the good times he could have, let him experience what he had to…

Speaking of Loz, where was he? He had let Dean know that he was going outside onto the smokers' veranda for a quick breather, but then that was almost twenty minutes ago.

'Loz?' Dean called, walking outside, the briskness in the air hitting him.

Loz was there, seemingly having a good time talking to a bunch of randoms - two guys and four girls - who were roaring with laughter at something he had apparently said.

'Heeey! Looky-look here, guys,' Loz squeaked, while walking unsteadily across the boards to Dean. He draped a heavy arm around him and leaned on him for support. 'This, everybody, is my very newest bestest best friend, Dean. Dean, everybody.' He threw his arms about him dramatically, as if conducting an orchestra.

Hi, guys.' Dean nodded, not slightly embarrassed.

They all smiled at him, acknowledging his presence, but then turned back to an earlier conversation between themselves.

Sensing they had been snubbed, Dean led Loz away. 'Friends of yours?' he grumbled, holding the drunken Loz up, who was now busying himself by searching for morsels of drink left over in discarded glasses on any tables they passed.

'Who?'

'The guys you were talking to just then,' Dean laughed.

'Nah. Di-you know 'em?' he slurred.

'Loz, you introduced them to *me*!'

'Ah sod 'em, then. They weren't very fun, anyway. Ooh, I love this song! Let's go dance some more!'

Before Dean knew it, he was being dragged back inside onto the dance floor and straight into a large group of hen party girls. The girls, however, didn't seem all that upset by the intrusion, and greeted Loz as if they had known him all their lives. They were, of course, as out of it as he was.

Once Dean was sure he wouldn't be missed, he took a step to the side and watched on, chuckling to himself. Loz was clearly having a whale of a time, hands in the air, jumping about. And it had to be said, he was quite the dancer, wiggling around as he did. People were virtually queuing up to dance with him, to get a piece of this new mover. He really was a curious one, this Laurence Price.

CHAPTER 7.

'Ow,' I whimpered.

I had woken up the next morning at home (thank God!), shoes off, and sprawled diagonally across my bed. It was 11:00am! - I had never slept in so late before. My throat felt like sandpaper, my head was pounding and my stomach was wrecked. I had never had such a combination of ailments at any one time in all my life, either. So this was what they called a "hangover!"

Just then, I noticed the mop bucket on the floor beside me, and I didn't need to look inside to know what was in it.

How had I got here? I literally couldn't think. I felt quite ashamed of myself, actually, for having let myself go so mad; it was so out of character. I tried to tally up how much I had drunk and gave up after the first six - not a good sign. And, unless Dad already knew, I certainly couldn't let him find out about it!

I had a quick shower, then subtly emptied the contents of the bucket down the toilet, and (once cleaned, of course) hid it under my bed out of sight – it would have looked far too suspicious if I breezily took it down stairs. I was trying my best to make everything seem as normal as possible - a very hard thing to do when you felt as though your internal organs were rotting from the inside out (another very new sensation I wasn't particularly fond of, and had only had the privilege of experiencing since knowing Dean).

'Good morning!' Dad said, half-amused, half-annoyed, as I entered the kitchen and made a beeline for the fridge for juice - I had a thirst on me akin to a third world person!

'The kitchen is now closed,' he said again with a mock smile, as he continued wiping down the surfaces. From the smell of things, everyone had just had a fry-up for brunch.

'I'm so sorry, Dad,' I managed between gulps, 'I didn't mean to, it just sort of happened, and, and then I guess I got kinda carried away, and...'

He just tutted and shook his head. 'It's okay. Just don't let it happen again, alright?'

That was unexpectedly lenient. '...Erm, okay?'

'You'll end up sleeping your whole day away, lying-in so late like that, and it's a waste. I just don't want you turning into one of those lazy teenagers. You know, the ones who doss around in life.'

So he didn't know after all.

'Oh, right, yeah. You're right, I'll try not to do it again.' I gave him a weak smile, and then headed straight for the cupboard under the stairs where the medicine box was kept. I was in serious need of some strong medication!

'By the way, have you seen the mop bucket at all?' Dad called after me. 'It seems to have gone walkies.'

An hour or so later, Dean came down. I had been sitting watching boring mid-Saturday TV in the living room waiting for him to show up, only too aware that we were being given a lift into town soon - not that I wanted to go much anymore, though. Part of me was on the brink of death, and the other part still felt hugely embarrassed about last night. I couldn't help but think that Dean had something to do with our getting safely home.

'Morning,' he said groggily, dragging his feet into the room. He did look rough, yet he managed to pull it off well enough.

'It's afternoon, actually,' I corrected.

'Oh, okay. Afternoon, then.'

Silence.

'The guys will be here at 2:00pm to pick us up,' he said, slumping into a chair.

''Kay.'

We were still going out, then.

Silence again, as Dean put his head back and began dozing sweetly. I watched him, entranced.

Just then, Dad and Bonnie strode in, wheeling Nana in her chair. Dean forced his eyes wide open, trying to make himself look as awake as possible.

'Right, lads. We're off to Ipswich. I promised I'd show Bonnie around, and Nana needs a few bits while we're there. You two gonna be alright?' Dad said, playing with his car keys.

'Fine. Absolutely fine.' Dean smiled falsely. 'Me and Loz will be meeting some mates in town later, so...'

'Okay, but don't be out late again, mind,' Bonnie told her son, wagging an authoritative finger.

'We won't, *mother*,' he sighed impatiently.

Once the front door had slammed behind them, Dean turned to me and said impishly, 'Bless 'em - clueless pair.'

I sat up properly. 'So they really don't know about last night?' I asked.

'Nope - they were sound asleep when we got back. Though I don't know how. You were making as much noise as you possibly could!'

I blushed hard. 'I'm sorry about that. Thanks for getting me home in one piece.'

'No problem. You just made me laugh, that's all. And you went proper wild in that club! Seriously, I've never seen a guy with so many girls on one dance floor in all my life. I think some of the lads in there were feeling a bit of the green-eyed monster; I certainly was!'

I suppose I had to laugh at myself. 'What happened with Donna?'

He shrugged. 'Nothing much. We kinda got separated in the club. She was getting on my nerves, to be honest - very clingy.'

Knowing that made me immensely happy, though I tried not to let it show. At least she was gone; she wouldn't be pestering him anymore!

'And how did we get back here?'

'The 3:00am late bus service. You were funny then, too - having a good ol' natter with this couple sitting in front of us, telling them about how the hose pipe ban this summer shouldn't have effected how much water we were allowed to use etc.' He snickered, rubbing his tired eyes.

I smacked my forehead, ashamed. God, I really was a hopeless case. I had definitely lost that very last shred of dignity I had been trying desperately hard to hold on to. I was amusing to Dean, but still a disaster. He would never be able to take me seriously.

'You're a class act, you are!' he chuckled, getting up and dragging his heels into the kitchen.

Randal - or Randy - and Harry picked us up at 2:00pm, as expected. I was quickly introduced, and then we were shoved into the back seats of the rather dirty-looking Peugeot 206, which you could tell was once a nice enough looking car before its present owner.

Dean and I had to squash in between the random bits and pieces that had accumulated on the seats; sports bags, football boots, dried mud, sweet wrappers and numerous empty drinks bottles just thrown back there out of the way and forgotten. It didn't smell too fresh, either.

'Sorry about the mess, dudes,' Randal said. Though I could tell he wasn't all that concerned for our comfort level; his mind was obviously on the road. I noticed, as well, that he wasn't wearing a seatbelt, and I contemplated how ready I felt about a road accident death. I didn't say anything, however - the self conscious part of me trying to suppress my nerdy outbursts. I wanted to stay in their good books, after all.

Dean was playing catch-up with Harry, who was sitting in the front passenger seat, letting him know all the gritty details of our adventures from the night before.

'Aw, man, you should have called us! Me and Randy would've been well up for it! Wouldn't we, mate?' he whined, prodding his friend annoyingly.

Randy swatted Harry's hand away. 'Yeah, definitely.'

Conversation then turned to me.

'So, tell us a bit more about your little pal, here, Deano,' Harry said, leaning round to get a closer look at me as if I was some strange phenomenon.

'He's called *Loz*, Harry. Don't patronise him; he has a mouth of his own, you know,' Dean chided.

'Well, so-rry!' he replied sarcastically. 'Fine, *Loz*, tell us a little about yourself.'

'Well, what do you want to know,' I asked dryly.

They both just 'um-med' and 'ah-ed.' I didn't honestly think they really wanted to know anything about me.

'You're in the same year as Jammy, aren't you? Friend of his?' Harry eventually said. Not that the question asked anything specific about *me*.

I just snorted rudely.

'I'll take that as a 'no,' then.' The front seat lads sneered at me. I wasn't sure how much I liked Dean's new friends.

'How long have you been driving, Randy?' I asked, steering the attention away from myself. I was curious, as surely Randy could have only just turned seventeen if he was, in fact, in Dean's year. How did he get his licence so quickly?

'About a year,' he said to my surprise.

'But--'

'I retook year twelve; I didn't do very well last year. I'm almost eighteen.'

Okay, so that made sense.

His apparent stand-offish nature and his inability to keep a clean car aside, Randy seemed to me to be the more preferable of the two. He was a freckly and lanky sort with auburn hair gelled into little spikes all over. He wore a mixture of fashions, taking a leaf out of both chav and emo books with his retro space invaders shirt and leather studded bracelets, matched with a pair of dowdy trackies and gaudy trainers. Now, I don't know fashion, but I was pretty sure that that was a bit of a no-no, and I couldn't say it looked right, either.

Harry, on the other hand, I didn't like one bit! He had a screwed up face, was quite badly acne-scarred and had an air of cockiness about him, which was always off-putting in anyone. I couldn't stand people who were up themselves. It was no wonder him and Jammy probably got on.

Once in town, we parked in the storey car park and made our way into the centre to meet up with Jammy and Cyndi. Apparently, Jammy had just finished a morning shift at his Saturday job and was free for the afternoon. Cyndi would be along later with a couple of her girlfriends - 'all ripe for the picking,' as Harry had so eloquently declared.

We found Jammy sitting outside Woolworths on a large concrete bench, smoking furiously, hugging his jacket tightly to him and looking about suspiciously, as though he was hiding something.

'Give it up, Jammy! Everyone knows you work at Woolies,' Harry shouted across the square to him as we drew near; he had been hiding his work shirt. Some people passing by looked about them nosily, wondering who the remark was directed at, and I almost felt a twinge of sympathy for him…almost.

'What's that thing doin''ere?' Jammy barked as he walked over to us, directing his annoyance with Harry at me.

Yep, definitely didn't sympathise with him *at all*!

That "thing," my dear James, is a *Loz*.' Dean said condescendingly, greeting his friend with a pat on the shoulder. 'I told you he was coming, didn't I? Besides, he's cool.'

I practically stumbled on the spot. He thought *I* was cool? I felt instantly smug.

Jammy scoffed back at him, 'He bloody well ain't!'

I snapped back. 'Don't worry, Jammy. I'm not exactly thrilled to be seen with you outside of school, either!'

'Whoa, check that dragon breathe!' Harry jeered, slapping me hard on the back so that it hurt. I would have clunked him round the back of the head in return if I had had the balls to.

'Hey! Leave the poor lad alone, guys,' Randy said, mercifully stepping in.

'Yeah! Come on, let's go get something to eat. My hangover's still got me starved!' Dean said, defusing the situation further and trying to move us on.

The afternoon was a warm one - one of the very few we had left before the Autumn properly kicked in - and we were walking around town with our chips-in-newspaper, wiling away the time before we met up with the girls.

At 3:30pm, we went to the park to wait for them. I was getting quite bored, to say the least. Harry and Randy were practically ignoring me, now; Jammy kept intimidating me with his sidelong glares at every opportunity he got; and Dean was doing his best to juggle between conversations with everyone, so it was no wonder he didn't have time to recognise my discomfort. I was tempted to just up and leave, do everyone a favour and get the bus back home and leave them all to it; I was clearly wasted space.

Eventually, Cyndi and her duo of luscious ladies tottered over to us. They were fashionably late, of course, and were wearing their most revealing summer clothes and fanciest sandals, trying to get as much use out of them as the lasting nice weather permitted. For the reactions they were undoubtedly after, it worked well.

The two other girls with Cyndi, I found out over a very giggly introduction, were called Zoë and Louise - both peroxide blonde bombshells (much like Donna had been), and like Cyndi, emitted sheer gorgeousness. Naturally, they all went down a treat with the guys, including Dean it seemed. That was all except me. I tried to pretend it was because I thought they were too OTT, when in actual fact I just wasn't attracted to them in the same way the others clearly were. They were beautiful, yes, but like a mantelpiece ornament is beautiful - you don't necessarily want to have sex with it!

'Ooh, look, girls! This is Loz. You remember? From my village?' said Cyndi, making her way through the mingling crowd to give me a big hug.

'Hi.' I staggered, choking slightly on a thick strand of her wavy hair. I wished she would get off of me.

'Oh, I'm so happy to see you out, honey! I never get to do anything with you, and I see you practically everyday. It's almost rude!' she exclaimed.

'Uh-huh.'

I felt totally misplaced. This was so not my scene. I missed Zen and Frankie - *my* people. These guys were far too cliquey and 2D for me, and for the first time, I was actually a little disappointed in Dean. I was even beginning to doubt my recent fixation with him. Was this *really* the kind of person he was? Part of me felt good about that, probably meaning my little crush thing was wearing off. But then I only had to look at him to realise that, sadly, that wasn't so.

'Ooh, we're gonna have fun today, just you wait!' she said, doing a little dance for me before moving over to jump on Dean.

Hello, jealousy!

I didn't have a fun day, contrary to what Cyndi thought. All they did was loiter and gossip about things only sixth formers were privy to. I was virtually forgotten, and so knowing that they were all very tempted to stay in town until late, drinking out in the pub beer gardens, I finally decided to take my cue to leave. I was still a little queasy from the adventures of last night, and felt it wise to steer clear of alcohol for a good while. Thankfully, the excuse worked. Dean and Cyndi put up a little fight, but they very quickly gave in as soon as the rounds were poured.

'You didn't enjoy yourself today, did you?' Dean said later that night when he came in.

It was 9:00pm, and I had been at my desk in my bedroom attempting some artwork.

'…It was…okay,' I answered unsurely. 'Did you not want to stay out later with them?'

'Nah, I'm shattered, so I got the bus back early,' he said, walking into the room and sitting on the end of my bed. Having him in my personal space felt very intimate. 'Listen, I guess I should have realised they wouldn't have been your kind of people. But I thought, what with Cyndi being there as well,…you know.'

'It's alright. I'm not blaming you for anything.' I smiled reassuringly at his splendid, but sorry-looking, face before the intensity of his gaze grew too much to bear and I turned away again.

'I'm sorry Harry and Randy weren't more accommodating, too. And Jammy!…' He tutted at the ceiling, 'You were right about him; he's really got it in for you!'

'You see?!'

'I wonder what his problem is?'

'You wouldn't be the first.'

He fidgeted a little where he sat. 'Look, they're okay most of the time - all of them, I mean. Honest. I know I've only known them for like a week, but they've been good to me.'

'Dean, don't worry about it. They're your friends, after all, not mine. Some people just don't mix.'

He thought about this. 'Yeah, I guess,' he sighed.

'Thanks for letting me come along, though,' I said, still smiling. 'I appreciated it all the same.'

'You're welcome.' He smiled back, then turned his attention to the opened sketchbook on my desk. 'What are you working on, there?'

'Art coursework,' I said apprehensively. I was outwardly very modest about my drawing skills, but inwardly I couldn't deny I had a flare.

'Can I look?' he asked, getting up and coming up beside me. I was wracked with nerves again.

'Err, well, it's not very good.' It really wasn't. I wasn't feeling especially motivated today and my talent was suffering.

'Let me be the judge of that. C'mon, move your hand,' he tittered at my reluctance, taking the book from my grasp.

He began to flick through, and almost instantly his eyes widened.

'Loz, these are awesome!'

My face burned. 'They're really not.'

'Don't be daft! Yes, they bloody well are!' he laughed. 'I'd kill to be able to draw like this! Why is it full of birds, though?'

'Erm,…that was my theme. The Swan.'

'Eh?'

'We had to select a theme from a list of random words and run with it - research it from all angles etc. - and I chose to do mine about The Swan.'

He still looked confused. 'But why *The Swan?*'

'I don't know, really. It was kind of an instinctive choice. They're quite impressive to look at, you know. You almost feel…well, unworthy, I guess, in their presence…' As I said this dreamily, I was looking up at Dean and became momentarily mesmerised, watching as he continued thumbing through my work book.

'Well, this is brilliant, mate. Seriously,' he said, gently putting it back down onto the desk.

'Thank you.' His approval meant more to me than the moon.

There was a moment's silence while he stared down at the paint-stained cover of the book, as if mentally digesting what he had just seen.

'Shit, just looking at that work makes me realise I've actually got a truck load of my own stuff to be getting on with. I best get going, dude,' he said a little distractedly. 'See you in a bit, though, yeah?'

'Oh, okay…Bye,' I called after him. I felt suddenly quite lonely.

I spent a while mulling over the day's activities, thinking about

Dean's friends. Then, missing my own and remembering they wanted me to meet up with them tomorrow, I ran for the phone and dialled Frankie's number in earnest.

CHAPTER 8.

As time began to fly by unnoticeably, my feelings for Dean, if possible, grew unbearably stronger with each passing day. Needless to say, I did not go out with him and his mates again, nor was I even invited. Not that I minded, of course, because Dean and I had soon developed our own, more exclusive, friendship group. Just he and I, and that suited me fine.

As I had originally anticipated, though, Dean didn't sit next to me much on the school bus anymore. He tended to go to the back with Cyndi and the other sixth formers he had recently befriended. This didn't bother me too much, however, as I knew he didn't like me any less. In any case, I would have him all to myself later at home.

My only problem now was trying to restrain myself whenever it was just the two of us alone. When we chatted together late in the evenings - me at my desk and Dean perched on the end of my bed, as was normal - about the day we had had, or about any school gossip that we had heard, I was constantly fighting back the urges to do all manner of unmentionable things to him. Whenever he spoke, or smiled, or laughed, I looked on in awe. I couldn't help but want to be close to him, to be able to touch him, to taste his cute little lips, while holding his perfect face in my hands and staring endlessly into his intoxicating eyes. And I wished so hard for him to want me to do it, too!

I thought of him all day, everyday, and at night I often dreamt of him. My crush was fast manifesting into something much more alarming than pure admiration, I knew that much. But the more comfortable I grew around him, the less I cared about his affect on me. Dean made me feel so lifted, that how could whatever it was I felt for him possibly do me any harm? I really loved being around him.

Even so, I wasn't stupid enough to say anything to anyone else about it. Could you imagine? They just wouldn't understand. No, I had resigned myself to believing that everything would sort itself out one day, for better or for worse. But as far as I was concerned, it didn't need to be dealt with at the moment. Why sort out today what you can put off 'til tomorrow? Or so the old saying goes.

On one particularly uneventful evening, Dean and I were up watching telly in my room. Predictably, there wasn't much on, so we settled on Wife Swap.

It was a fairly typical episode this week. One woman was a council estate super slag with six kids under ten, all of whom had different dads. Her most recent husband had only really known her two months and she already had baby number seven in the oven!

The second woman was a high-powered career mum, whose husband, much like herself, was barely around to see their, now relatively independent, eleven-year old daughter. Personally, I couldn't help but feel sorry for all of the kids involved. I guess I had to count myself lucky. Even though my mum was no longer around, at least she *had* been there for me when she was alive.

'This is crap!' Dean groaned.

'Do you want to switch over...?'

'Can't we just turn it off?'

I did as he suggested; the show was starting to bore me, too. I didn't know what we would do instead, though.

'What was your mum like?' Dean blurted out of the blue, sitting himself up attentively as if ready to be regaled.

'...Oh, erm.' He really had caught me a little off guard. 'Well,...a bit like me...Or so I'm told.'

'Hmm.' He pondered this.

'...But *I* don't believe that. I mean, she really was something special,' I said, beginning to reminisce.

I never spoke much about my mum. Although it had been six years since her death, the memory of her could still pull me apart whenever I was feeling especially fragile. Another factor was that I didn't like how people pried. As far as I was concerned, she was nobody else's business but mine. But for some reason, in Dean's encouraging presence, I felt the need to open up - I actually *wanted* to talk to him about her. Memories once kept at bay by immense willpower, now flooded my mind as fresh as ever. It suddenly mattered to me that Dean should know about this extraordinary person, who had then been so unfairly wrenched away from me. It was as if by telling him about her was, in a way, giving him a part of myself, and since I couldn't give him a lot else, that would just have to suffice.

'I've been told that, apparently, I'm the spitting image of her. But I only have to look back at her photos to know that they're lying. She was really beautiful,' I continued confidently. 'She had a smile that could melt butter - or at least that's how my dad puts it.'

I reached over to my bedside table and opened the drawer. Tucked neatly in the corner was a small picture frame containing my favourite picture of Mum - her sitting out in the sun eating an ice cream and looking out over our garden. The picture was surprisingly well taken, considering it had been taken with the little plastic My First camera that I had been given for my 8th birthday. She had died the following year.

I delicately handed Dean the frame. 'This is her.'

He stared at her. 'She *is* beautiful,' he said, smiling. 'She does look a lot like you, too.'

I looked at him curiously for a moment. But then finally choosing to ignore the subtle compliment, I carried on talking. The words were coming easily to me now, as if I said them all the time.

'She was always so happy.' I beamed. 'But she had a laugh that could crack a window pane!

'She and Dad ran this place together, and everyday was like living with a real life Snow White. Life was never dull. She would sing and dance around all the time, turning everything into a game.

'I remember one time - when I was about five or six - it was raining outside and business was slow, and I was bored. So, Mum decided it would be fun to get out some old bed sheets and pull all the living room furniture together to make an imaginary pirate ship - we used the ironing board as a plank.' I snickered. 'I pretended I was Peter Pan, and Mum played both Captain Hook and Wendy.

We ended up having a sword fight using recycled cardboard box flaps.'

I laughed at the crystal clear memory of how silly and fun it had been, and then sobered at the thought of how long ago it was. 'It's not an amazing memory, I know, but it's one that sticks with me,' I said glumly.

But Dean just smiled sweetly, glancing up at me. 'That sounds like a perfect memory to me.'

His dazzling face, mixed with my own sense of renewed grief for my mum, was proving a little too much to take all at once. I looked away from him and inconspicuously wiped away a tear.

'You must miss her,' he said gently.

I turned to him. But the look on my face must have been enough to say it all, as another betraying tear rolled slowly down my cheek.

He looked horrified. 'Oh, God, Loz! I'm sorry, mate. I shouldn't have--'

He then moved over to sit close to me. By his hesitant gestures, I could tell he wanted to comfort me, but didn't seem entirely sure how to go about it. In the end, he settled for putting a loose arm around me, hugging me slightly, and calmingly rubbing my forearm.

Despite myself, my heart raced and my skin went all goosepimply.

'No, no. It's fine, honestly. I'm just being silly. It was all such a long time ago. I'm just not used to talking about her much, that's all.'

'I'm sorry, Loz,' he said again.

I dried my dampened face with my sleeve and grinned back at him. 'Don't be. You're the first person I've said all this to in a long time - it probably does me good.'

I then became very aware of how close he was. He was leaning a little into me, and he looked transfixed for a moment.

'Thank you,' I muttered, finding myself being equally drawn to him.

'Sure,' he replied softly.

He then blinked a couple of times and got up quickly, announcing that, regrettably, he needed to get to bed. He left just as hastily as he had the last time, and as always, I was left ever more hungry for him.

CHAPTER 9.

It was the first week in October, Wednesday lunchtime, and I had managed to drag Zen and Frankie out onto the windy sidelines of the playing field. Today was the first really cold day we had had since May – an indication of worse to come, no doubt.

'Why are we out here, Loz? It's freezing and you hate football,' Zen pouted, his hands in his parker jacket pockets and his mane blowing wildly this way and that. Wednesday lunchtimes were for the Sixth Form Cup matches. Both sixth form years split themselves into five-aside football teams, and each week two of the many amateur teams battled it out. The losing team would be inevitably thrown out of the tournament. This would carry on until the finals in December, so there was a way to go, but then there were a lot of teams in the league to get through.

And yes, though I did indeed hate football, this week was Dean's team, the year 12 Guerrillas', first match against the year 13 Tossers - a name apparently very fitting for the players of which the team consisted, according to Dean - and I had promised to make a special effort to show my support. Not that I had needed much persuading, though.

'I told Dean I'd be here for him, Zen.'

'But why?' he moaned.

'Because he's, you know, a friend. And this is what friends do.'

'You guys are *friends*?' Frankie asked, surprised. 'Really?'

Her remark annoyed me at once. '*Yeah*! Why, is that so difficult to believe? We do live together, as well, you know.'

'I know, it's just…' she started.

'Go on,' I said crossly.

Why shouldn't Dean and I be friends? I mean, yes, I still had to pinch myself every now and then whenever I thought about how lucky I was to even know him and, much more, that he even liked me; but I just didn't like that others were just as baffled.

What Frankie said next, though, got me thinking.

'Well, it's just that you guys clearly run in totally different social circles. You're both so different.'

'We're not,' I maintained, though I didn't sound so sure of myself.

'Honestly, hon, it really doesn't matter what we--'

'Look, are you threatened by him?' I snapped irrationally. Though, really, I was just worried that she might have been right in some way. I instantly regretted it, in any case.

'Err, oi! Where did that come from?'

'Pfff, yeah, don't flatter yourself, mate!' Zen joked.

I looked away to breathe. I knew I was being very silly, now. They were my best friends and were, after all, standing out in the cold for me. And besides, *I* knew that Dean and I got on, irrespective of what anyone else thought. But I still felt that Zen and Frankie hadn't really given him a chance. I was convinced no-one could possibly dislike him, and I just wanted them to see what I saw.

'I'm sorry,' I said, quietly ashamed. 'But Dean's nice, guys. You shouldn't prejudge him. He's not like others.'

Frankie's expression softened. 'Fine, we'll take your word for it,' she sighed, giving me a playful shove.

I smiled weakly. 'You know you're my main crew, right?' Compulsion forced me to reassure them, even though I knew nothing had changed.

'Shut-up!' Zen chuckled.

'Yeah, shush, you, and watch your friend out there,' Frankie said, resting her chin on my shoulder.

At half time, Dean came over, panting, sweating and looking altogether quite smouldering with a well deserved grin on his face. It had been him who had scored most of the team's goals so far.

'Your doing well,' I called over to him.

'Thanks. And thanks for coming to watch.'

'Sure thing.' My mouth began to water as my eyes flitted about him distractedly, taking him all in and scanning for his every visible bulge.

'So, how many goals is it you guys have scored?' Zen interrupted. He had about as much of an idea of how to play the game as I did. To tell the truth, I hadn't really been watching any of it, either - more so Dean, admiring his athletic body prancing majestically around the pitch - but I still at least knew that his team was winning.

'It's 5:1 to us,' Dean breathed while stretching his limbs.

'Ah, well…you're doing great, then. Like Loz said,' Frankie added. Football wasn't an easy conversation starter for her, either.

'Cheers.' He nodded before turning back to me, 'You know, if you guys are getting too cold, you don't have to stay. I understand it's not really your thing.'

'No, no, we'll stay,' I said, perhaps a little too eagerly. 'I said I would.'

'Okay, well, I'm gonna go grab a quick drink and catch up with the others. Enjoy the rest, if you can.' He smiled at us as he turned and jogged his way further down the sidelines to where a huge posse - largely consisting of sixth form girls, including Cyndi - waited excitedly for him.

I stared after him longingly, and I must have been doing it a while, because pretty soon Frankie started tugging at my arm.

'Hon, are you okay?' she asked, catching my eye.

'Huh?' I snapped out of my trance. 'Oh, yeah…definitely.'

She just looked quizzically at me, searching my face for something.

The next lesson after lunch was P.S.H.E., and, like so many others, it was not one of my favourites. This was primarily because I had to put up with Jammy for a whole hour! - most lessons only lasted forty-five minutes or so.

As was routine, Jammy would no doubt find it virtually impossible to refrain from verbally abusing me in front of the class. He also always made a point of sitting as close to me as possible in order to do so, as well. I didn't even have Zen or Frankie to stick up for me - they weren't in any of the classes I shared with Jammy.

The teachers were practically useless, too! They could barely look after themselves, fending off thirty or so disobedient and hormonally driven teens, let alone save me from Jammy's relentless harassment! So far, I wasn't doing very well at avoiding him this year.

I didn't like to moan too much to Dean about Jammy, either, as I didn't want him to think of me as anymore of a drip than I probably already was in his eyes. I had to learn to fight my own battles.

'Right, then,' said Mrs Tchaikovsky to the unruly class that afternoon in the draughty hut. 'Today, we're going to look at *sexuality*.'

'Gay boys!' an immature prick in the back row heckled, causing most of the class to giggle uncontrollably.

'Enough!' Mrs Tchaikovsky bellowed, silencing everyone. 'But yes, the word *gay* does obviously come into play.'

'Your kind of lesson, then. Eh, Pricey?' Jammy sneered at me, his band of merry morons smirking along with him. Each of them gave me a slap on the back and pushed me about in my seat. I tried to ignore them. If I wasn't such a goody-two-shoes in front of teachers, I would have definitely given them a few choice words to think over!

'Settle down, boys!' the teacher said dismissively. 'Now, *sexuality*, as you are no doubt all aware, is a strong, physical and mental attraction to someone…or something.'

She turned and wrote two separate, almost illegible, words in cursive hand writing on the blackboard: *Heterosexuality and Homosexuality* - two of my least favourite words these days. Why did they have to be so categorised like that?

'Now, I'm going to try not to insult your intelligence, but I have to know that you understand the meaning of these two very common terms.'

'*Heterosexuality* is when you fancy someone of the opposite sex, Miss,' Julie Riggs called out, her hand shot fast in the air and not even waiting to be asked.

Everyone groaned. Julie was the queen of swots. I only fell into the minor swot category, but if there had to be a land full of swots, she would definitely be ruler of them all.

'Oh, why don't you just go kiss her arse, Julie!' someone hissed.

Julie obviously heard it, but pretended otherwise, still looking happy at her contribution.

'That's right. Thank you, *Julie*,' Mrs Tchaikovsky said, glaring about the room, looking for the nasty culprit before eventually giving up and turning to write down the description underneath the obscurely written *Heterosexuality*. 'Though next time, please don't shout out, Julie.'

The class laughed triumphantly at her and, this time, Julie did go red.

'The next one, anyone?'

'Please, Miss?' Jammy pleaded.

'Yes, James?'

'*Homosexuality* is people like my mate, Pricey, here. They like it up the bum!'

Everyone roared with laughter, except for me. Like Julie before me, I had gone crimson, feeling a mixture of intense embarrassment and seething rage. How come I was the sudden butt of gay jokes?

Mrs T. was furious. 'James, that was highly inappropriate and totally uncalled for! You're on your second warning--'

'But I've not even had my first!' he complained.

She ignored him. 'One more and it's straight to the Head's office! Do you understand?'

He muttered, 'yes,' and leaned back sulkily in his chair. But as soon as Mrs T. resumed teaching, he turned to me and grinned widely like a Cheshire cat, showing absolutely no signs of remorse. One of his oaf-like drones, Eddy Collier, leant across me, deliberately making a mess of my work space, to give his friend an approving nudge. I stared venomously at them both, but they just pulled stupid faces back at me.

'Can anyone *sensible*,' Mrs T. stressed, purposely looking over at Jammy and pointing at the board, 'tell me the meaning of this word?'

'Miss?'

'Anyone besides Julie?'

'Miss! Miss!'

'Come on, this is unbelievably easy!' She knew we all knew the answer, it's just that nobody except Julie - and Jammy, apparently - could be bothered to answer, lest they be mistaken for a bookworm.

'Someone who's attracted to members of the same sex, Miss.' Julie blurted out, unable to control herself any longer.

'God, you're such a geek, Julie!' Nina Stoppard whispered loudly in the corner with the rest of the Max Factor ensemble.

'Thank you.' Mrs T. had obviously given up on keeping Julie in check. It was no use, as hard as all the teachers tried. It was like she was afflicted with some sort of OCD to please, but ironically for her, the teachers all secretly hated her for it.

'Now, your sexuality is nothing to be ashamed of. It is perfectly natural to fall for people of either your own sex or the opposite, and sometimes even both. Can someone tell me what I mean by that that last part? Nina?'

'Bisexuality, Miss,' she said half-heartedly before blatantly yawning.

'Yes, that's right.' Mrs T. wrote some more on the board behind her. 'Sometimes, sexuality can be very confusing - at your age especially, with hormones pulsating through you all the time. And so, a common worry is having homosexual desires or tendencies. Some people are known to go through what are occasionally referred to as "gay phases," and temporary crushes on friends or role models of the same sex are more common than you might think - it doesn't necessarily mean you're gay. Having said that, there is absolutely nothing wrong with it if eventually you do find yourself more that way inclined...'

Throughout the rest of Mrs T.'s lecture, I was increasingly aware of how intently people were beginning to listen...for a change. I suddenly felt more at ease with myself, thinking of the many people in my own class who had possibly experienced, or were experiencing, similar emotions as me.

It was, therefore, a relief to know that, on some level, I wasn't alone. I was by no means a *freak*, as I had once thought - I could see that now.

However, what it also made me finally realise, was that I no longer wanted my feelings for Dean to change. Not ever.

CHAPTER 10.

Later that same evening…

'Loz? It's Frankie.'

'Oh, hey!' I took the upstairs portable phone into my room and closed the door. 'What's up?'

'Erm, not a lot.'

'No?'

'No,' she said.

There was a pause.

I laughed. 'Then, why are you calling?'

'Why, can't a girl ring a friend for an unscheduled chinwag whenever she wants?' she said, sounding slightly affronted.

'Frankie!'

'Okay, okay…There is something.'

'Uh-huh?'

'It's about earlier…'

'What?'

'…Look, it's not easy for me to come out with this, so here goes…' she said. There was another brief pause, which unnerved me. 'Are you, you know,…*okay?*'

'I'm fine.' I answered quickly. 'Why?'

'Well, you just seem a bit…*off* recently, that's all.'

'What do you mean by "off ?" Since when?'

'Since Dean.'

Silence.

My heart rate immediately quickened, and I took in a long, erratic breath. I knew exactly what she was driving at.

'There's nothing wrong with me, Frankie. Thanks for checking up on me, I appreciate it, but there's absolutely nothing to worry about,' I lied in my firmest voice.

'Hon, it's okay. You can tell me. I'm your best friend and I won't say anything to anyone, not even Zen if that's what you want--'

'There's nothing to say.'

'But Loz--'

'Seeya tomorrow, Frankie,' I said sternly before punching the receiver-down button and pushing the phone as far away from me on the desk as possible.

My hands shook violently.

She was on to me like a fox, but I still wanted to play dumb for a while longer. She *was* my best friend, though, and I did feel guilty for not confiding. But then, what exactly would I say? 'Hi, Frankie! Yes, I am secretly head-over-heels for some random who lives with me, and who I've known for little more than a month. Oh, and to top it off, he's a *guy*, and one who's totally out of my league, for that matter!' The thought of even saying those exact words was enough to make me want to be sick; it scared me. I felt so much better when I wasn't analysing things.

Just then, I heard a rap at the door and in walked Dean.

My anxieties miraculously disappeared in a heartbeat, and I practically forgot all about the conversation I had had with Frankie only minutes before. Dean lit up the room and dazzled me like he always did. 'Hi,' I sighed.

'Hey, dude.' he said warmly, coming in and setting himself down with his books. My insides were all gooey.

As scheduled, he had come to study with me. We both had Maths tests this week, so taking heed of his example, I got out my own books and got to work.

After a gruelling one-hour session poured over revision guides, we decided to take a break. I put the radio on to help us unwind; the Scott Mills show played distantly in the background.

'God, I hate Maths!' I heaved, collapsing back onto the bed. My head hurt already.

I felt rather guilty, as I had needed Dean's help a lot over my numerous algebra problems, having to interrupt him from his own studying. But he assured me that it was just as useful for him, too, being able to go back over the basics of his own work.

'Meh, it's not so bad.' He shrugged, stretching out his legs on the bed. He was sat at the opposite end to me

I wondered for a moment, the beat of the music echoing gently around me. 'Dean? Do you think we're too...*different*?'

He was visibly taken aback. 'What? Why do you say that?'

'People have been pointing it out to me, that's all.'

He raised an eyebrow 'By "people," do you mean Zen and Frankie?'

'Well,...kind of,' I said more meekly.

'Why do they say we're so different, then?'

'It's fairly obvious, don't you think?'

He shook his head at me. 'I don't think so. Tell me,' he demanded. He sounded noticeably hurt.

'Well, you like sports,...' - Girls - '*Maths*!...' I struggled.

He looked mildly relieved by my pitiful attempt. 'That's all you've got? That's just skin deep stuff – it's nothing.'

I tutted. 'It's not just that, though. I mean, look at us! I'm a weedy school boffin, and you're a cool, confident, funny, smart, kind, caring, good-looking--'

Dean laughed, interrupting my seemingly endless flow of compliments. 'I think I'm in danger of being overly flattered.'

'But it's all true,' I said bashfully.

His face suddenly grew understanding. 'So, really, you're basing our so called "differences" on our popularity at school.'

I begun to see why that sounded so silly, but still I persisted. I just couldn't see why someone as extraordinarily wonderful as him would want to bother with someone as dull and plain as me - not that my looks would be of any consequence to him either way, of course.

'It *does* make a difference, Dean.' My tone was rueful.

He frowned. 'Hey! Weren't *you* the one who told *me* once that some people just don't mix?'

Did he just quote *me*? I had to think back hard to remember my own words, though. What was he getting at? 'Yeah, I suppose--'

'But that's not always the case, is it?' he continued.

I was still confused. 'What?'

'Loz, just because we run in slightly different social circles at school doesn't mean we can't otherwise get on. As it is, I find *you* rather cool, confident - in your own way - and I think you're funny - you're always making me laugh. You're also amazingly talented, though tirelessly modest about it; you're kind, considerate, and I certainly don't think you're "weedy." Take it from me, you're a good-looking kid, too.'

I could feel my cheeks burning. I really was far too modest to believe any of this.

Just then, however, my newest favourite song came on the radio.

'Aw, tune! Metro Station!' Dean's voice echoed in my head. He pretended to dance while still sitting cross-legged on the bed.

I had to laugh at him.

'You like Metro Station?' I was surprised. He didn't seem like the type who was into alternative music.

'Of course!' He snorted. 'Don't you?'

'Err,…hell, yeah!' I cried above the lyrics. I then dived into the song, humming the verses I didn't know.

This seemed to amuse him, as well. 'Funny. I never would have figured you'd be into this kind of alternative stuff,' he said.

I smiled at the irony. 'Are you kidding me? I love it! Maybe not so much the hardcore stuff, but I like Alphabeat, The Killers, Coldplay…'

'They are pretty cool bands.' He nodded, and then chuckled to himself.

'What?'

'And you said you didn't think we had anything in common!' he teased, throwing a pillow at me.

I giggled and threw it back at him. What ensued was a very uneven pillow fight, as Dean managed to almost knock me off the bed with his almighty whopping strength. He caught me just as I went flying, though, accidentally pulling me back on top of him.

The laughter quickly died, and we just stared at each other in shock, me lying across him. His sheer proximity, mixed with the feeling of his hard body beneath mine, was enough to make me go all woozy. I had to remember to mentally jump start my heart again when I realised I wasn't breathing anymore. Neither of us said a word.

Then, reminding myself that I was, indeed, still in his lap, I hastily got up and scrambled my way back to my books.

'I suppose we ought to get some more work done,' I stuttered, breaking the awkward silence. My hands were trembling as they fumbled for my notes.

Quiet again.

Dean cleared his throat. 'Let me know if you need anymore help with that.'

I didn't look at him as I answered, 'Yeah, thanks,' and turned back to the unsolved equations that vied for my attention.

CHAPTER 11.

A week later, on Friday evening, after I could no longer make up anymore excuses not to see her, I went back with Frankie to her house after school. I really hadn't been looking forward to the idea ever since she mentioned it the day after our little phone conversation about Dean - she had been good enough to not mention anything to Zen, at least. In the end, however, I convinced myself that the opportunity to confront her meant that I would be able to warn her to drop the subject once and for all.

Once inside her house, she led me up the small flight of stairs to her bedroom and closed the door. Her room was brilliant; it was filled with quirky bits and pieces ranging from the lava lamp bedside lamp and the glow in the dark dinosaur stickers from her tomboyish childhood, which were now permanently glued to the tired looking door, to the retro disco ball that hung from the ceiling. Her walls were literally covered with bands of all genres, too, so much so that there wasn't even the slightest hint of wallpaper - the posters were the wallpaper!

Frankie's parents weren't in, and her older sister, Katie, though safely out of our way in her room, was listening to her pounding punk / rock music on the highest possible volume setting. You could hear the harsh thud-thud of the baseline pumping its way through every wall of the small, three-bedroom council estate house. It sounded like there was an elephant's party going on, and everything about us vibrated. Frankie banged away on her side of the wall until Katie finally gave in and cooperated.

'I don't know why I bother sometimes, you know. She'll only turn it back up again in a minute.'

Sure enough, after a few minutes or so - or once Katie had eventually decided that there had been sufficient quiet time - the noise went right back up again.

'She better bloody turn it down soon, or else the neighbours will be round moaning again!' Frankie growled. 'And she'll be taking the heat for it this time, not me!'

She went about the room grumbling to herself, and putting objects that had been knocked down by the vibrating walls back in their rightful places.

'Frankie…' I called out to her. The racket next door was distracting and I wanted to sort things out now so that I could go home.

'Hmm?' she mumbled loudly, not really paying attention. I knew she was used to all this and I didn't honestly think she really minded the noise all that much, just that it got the family into so much trouble around the estate. But of all the times I had been here I had *never* got used to it, and, therefore, always tried to hint that we would probably be better off at either mine or Zen's.

'Let's step out for a bit,' I suggested, 'The noise is doing my head in.'

The day was another unusually warm one, so we decided to go and sit out on the village green. Frankie's village, Little Wiggan, was pretty unspectacular. It was about two villages north of mine, and, technically, I could walk the distance, but it would still take me a good half an hour. Unfortunately for her, Frankie didn't live in the most privileged part of the village; her road was full of chavvy, street-wise, white-trash families. But the green was a little way down the road from all that - at the "nicer end" - and bar a few kids kicking a football around, the area was near enough deserted.

'This is nice. I didn't think I'd be able to do this again for a while,' she sighed blissfully, sprawled out in front of me and pointedly picking up a few dried leaves from off the ground around her. 'What with the leaves falling, and all.'

It was true, the seasons were finally turning for good. We had been blessed with a long and beautiful summer, but now, in mid October, it really was time for the rest of the autumn leaves to begin their long overdue floating decent to the ground.

'Yeah,' I said dismissively, no longer interested in conversational pleasantries. 'Frank, why have you been so insistent on seeing me?'

She gawped at me with a look of false hurt.

'Can't a girl see her best friend when she wants to without there being a real reason?'

I suppressed a smirk. 'Cut the crap, Frank!'

'Oh, alright, alright…' she huffed. 'I needed to talk to you face to face about this, but you've been pretty good at avoiding me lately.'

'What? I have not!' I argued, though I knew she was right. Each time I had seen her that week, I made sure she was followed by Zen first before going over. In the end, being unsuccessful in getting me to herself, she started ringing me up at least five / six times a day. After a load of lame excuses, I was soon all out, and so reluctantly gave in to her.

'You have too! I saw you scarper the other day when you saw me down the hallway coming out from the languages department. I called out to you and you just ignored me. Then later at lunch, when Zen was around, you acted as if nothing had even happened!'

I could see from her flushed cheeks that she was quite miffed. There was an awkward pause.

'I'm sorry if I gave you that impression,' I said quietly.

'Why won't you talk to me, Loz? I feel like I don't know you these days. Both me *and* Zen have noticed a change in you.'

'I haven't changed, and there's nothing to talk about,' I lied, fidgeting.

'See, I just know there is. Come on, tell me.'

I snapped. 'Frankie, why do I *have* to tell you? You're my friend, yes, but exactly *why* do I have to tell you? If there *was* anything the matter - which there isn't – did you ever stop to think it might be something embarrassingly personal? I mean, for all you know, it could be something that I don't even know how to properly admit to myself, let alone--'

'I know it's Dean, Loz.'

Her words stunned me, stopping me mid-flow. '…Except it isn't.'

'Do you fancy him, Loz?' she asked bluntly.

And there it was, the very question I had dreaded hearing out loud.

My heart beat a hundred times its normal pace. 'What?'

'Do you,' she said again more slowly, 'fancy Dean?'

'Look, just because Dean lives with me, and just because we're friends, it doesn't mean I--'

'I've seen the way you are around him. I know the signs, hon. Trust me,' she said gently, placing a comforting hand over mine. I flinched.

'I, I...' I couldn't think of what else to say. My mind had gone blank. In spite of having told myself earlier to deny whatever accusations Frankie threw at me, it was getting increasingly harder the more persistent she became.

'Please tell me, hon. I won't think any less of you, I promise. You know I'll still love you no matter what,' she said in hushed tones, looking probingly into my eyes with her own. 'Don't hide.'

Her words were heartfelt, and they instantly struck a chord with me. All kinds of emotions from the past month or so started to stir within me. My eyes began to fill, and I quickly turned my head to blink away the tears, hoping she hadn't seen. But before I knew it, she was right by my side with an arm around my shoulder, rocking me. My eyes leaked unrelentingly, the tears soaking into her cardigan as I broke down.

'It's okay, babe,' she soothed understandingly, giving my shoulder a squeeze and resting her chin on the top of my head. 'It's perfectly okay,' she said again.

We sat there for a long time not talking, waiting for my tear ducts to dry up.

'Look,' she started after a minute, 'I promise you I'm not going to say anything to anyone. But listen, it really doesn't matter to me who or what you are, and I'm sure it wouldn't matter to anyone else. If ever you want someone to talk to, though, you know I'm always here.' She gave me a big, comforting smile and one last squeeze before moving away from me.

The thing is, I wasn't really all that upset about her finally finding me out, despite my previous concerns. In fact, I was a little relieved that I didn't have to deal with whatever was going on inside me all on my own - I wasn't suffering so much anymore; it had been an exhausting burden to bear alone. But what really upset me, and what was the real reason for my tears, was realising that not only was I interested in a *guy*, but that I was also interested in a guy who couldn't have been more straight. Talk about unrequited! It was gut-wrenching, and it hurt *a lot* - a kind of heartache in itself, knowing that I would never be wanted by the one person I wanted more than I had ever wanted anything before. It was so unfair, that the stress and realisation of it all caused a melt down.

After a little more time had passed, I then bravely admitted, if somewhat numbly, 'I think I'm in love with him, Frank.'

Her expression didn't change as she took in what I said. 'Are you sure it's not *just* a crush, Loz?'

I shook my head. 'No.' I said decisively. And having said it out loud only made it feel all the more real. 'I *love* him.'

And that was it; I had undergone the seemingly irrevocable transformation - I was in love. Dean excited me, through and through, and no-one I had ever known in my whole life could compare. And no-one, I was certain, ever would.

CHAPTER 12.

October 24th was a very special day. It was a Saturday, but it was also Dean's birthday, and I was incredibly excited for him. He was now seventeen.

I had spent the evening before helping Nana to bake the cake, while Dean was out round one of his friends' houses. Bonnie was quite set on doing it herself, but Nana wouldn't hear of it, having to practically fight her off out of the kitchen with the ends of her walking sticks. Nana may not have been the best cook, but she loved to bake. At any rate, Dad had in mind - as a rather convenient distraction - to take Bonnie to see a film.

I, at least, *was* allowed to help Nana. Dad had refused to totally leave her to her own devices in the kitchen - she was, after all, a liability! So, I promised him I would keep an eye on her, which was actually code for: 'I'll make sure she doesn't confuse the slug pellets for chocolate sprinkles again.'

I honestly didn't mind, though. I actually really wanted to help, and in the end, we baked him a very sturdy-looking - and hopefully edible - Victoria sponge with a layer of thick, white icing and 'Happy 17th Dean!' written in blue. Originally, I had thought about going for something a bit more adventurous, like an upside down cake, or maybe even a totally alternative take on birthday cakes altogether in the form of a soufflé. But then neither me or Nana were exactly professional pastry chefs, so I decided not to push our luck on that score. I was pretty sure Dean would like whatever we made him, anyway.

I made a point of going out to town on my own the weekend before to buy his card and present, too. I didn't want to presume too much, as I had only known him a short while. So, going by what I already knew about him, I spent the whole day hunting for the ideal gift. Unfortunately, I had very little pocket money, and so thought that to enable me to maximise my spending on the perfect present, I would economise on the card and make him one, instead. However, in spite of my creative mind, I wasn't the most imaginative gift buyer (both Zen and Frankie could vouch for that), but I figured that so long as I at least had a decent card, surely the present wouldn't matter as much. It was the thought that counted after all, right?

The thought of what to buy him had driven me near enough insane. I had to be careful that whatever I did buy didn't make me come across as an overly eager loser in desperation to impress a new friend - I didn't want to scare him away with overindulgence. In the end, I played it safe and bought him a Metro Station poster and a big bar of Cadbury's Dairy Milk. Again, nothing special, but I promised myself that I would make the card something that would really capture his attention.

Once home, I immediately got to work. And I carried on working every night of the week after school. All in all, I made five possible outcomes, but then I had the inevitably difficult task of whittling them down to just one. They were all fairly similar in that they were handcrafted with doodles of cars, footballs and an assortment of your typical party decorations, but I still wasn't overly impressed with my workmanship. They didn't have the *wow* factor I was aiming for. However, before I could even consider attempting a sixth version, I found it was already the following Friday, and so other preparations took precedence.

The next morning, on Dean's actual birthday, I got up especially early with the intention of giving him his present on my own. I wanted him for myself, to bask in his reactions.

I washed and dressed, and with gifts and card ready in hand, I tiptoed across the landing to his door and rapped lightly, calling his name in a low hiss, 'Dean! You awake?'

No answer.

I knocked and asked again, though this time a little louder.

'Um?' came a croaky voice.

I opened the door slightly. The oddly appealing, gentle musk of his room drifted out and found my nostrils, tempting me forwards.

'It's Loz,' I whispered from the other side, holding my ground. What if he was naked, I wondered. I had to fight an overpowering desire to not burst in.

'Um, huh?...Wh-what time is it?' the voice asked.

'7:30am.'

'What day is it?'

'Saturday.'

'Saturday?'

'Yeah.'

'Then,…why are we up?' he groaned.

'It's your birthday,' I answered matter-of-factly.

'So?'

'Don't you want your presents?'

Silence.

'Alright, come in.'

I sniggered as I entered. I hadn't been in Dean's room much, since he always tended to come to mine. But then, compared to his, I supposed my room did look a lot cosier; it was more lived in, like how a teenager's room ought to be.

I shuffled over to the window to open the curtains. The striking early morning sun immediately lit up the, once gloomy-looking, room.

Dean's room really wasn't anything fancy; it was only a guest bedroom - all white walls, brown carpeting and old, antique furnishings. And despite the fact that the Mackellars had been with us for a month and a half, now, there were still a fair few labelled, unpacked boxes scattered across his floor. Other than a portable telly at the foot of his bed, resting on top of an empty upside down box, and an ipod speaker system set up next to a book and his watch on the bedside table, there really wasn't much else to look at...save Dean. Everything was kept to a minimum; no real sense of personalisation. I guessed he had resisted the temptation to unpack fully, thinking that there was no point in doing so when he and his mum weren't planning on staying for very much longer.

My mood soured considerably when I thought about that. Bonnie and Dean were only booked up until the end of November. Then they would be out of here to wherever. I knew they would only end up moving somewhere nearby, but I couldn't bear the thought of Dean leaving. In the short time that he had been here, he had made a seemingly irreversible impression on me, and at least with him living with me I still had a kind of hold on him, not matter how tenuous. When he did eventually leave, though, he would no doubt drift away from me and I would be powerless to stop it. I shivered a little at that and decided not to allow myself to think about it. Today would be a happy day. Today was Dean's day.

'So, what you got for me, then?' he yawned, stretching and rubbing his eyes. He was still lying in bed with his sheets around him. For my heart's sake, I was glad he was wearing a T-shirt.

'You'll just have to wait and see, won't you.'

I grabbed the wooden chair from up against the far wall and pulled it close to him. I gazed at his half-asleep face for a second and loved what I saw. Even at his most undignified, he still managed to smoulder. I had to resist the temptation to clamber under the covers with him.

He pulled himself up, leaning his back against the, now upright, pillow. 'You really didn't have to bother, you know. I wasn't expecting anything.'

I handed him his gifts. 'Oh, really? Could have saved myself some cash, then, couldn't I?' I teased.

He smirked at me, then commenced tearing open the wrapping paper.

'Happy Birthday, by the way,' I said quickly before he was done.

'Thanks.' He beamed, revealing the bar of chocolate.

'It's nothing special, I know, but--'

'Nah! You can never go wrong with chocs.' He winked at me. 'Now, I wonder what this one could possibly be...'

I flushed at the note of sarcasm in his voice as he reached for the rather obvious poster-shaped present, but I was glad to see the same amused expression was still there on his face.

'Metro Station - wicked!'

'I thought you might need something to liven up these walls,' I justified.

'Aw, I love it! Thanks, mate.' His expression was wholly appreciative and I revelled for a moment in his raptures.

'Don't forget the card,' I pointed out.

Out of the five I had initially created, I was forced to choose the only one that was, I thought, halfway decent. It was a jokey / pop-up-type card that had taken me all of two evenings to make. Needless to say, I was thoroughly behind in my homework.

He carefully tore open the handmade envelope and pulled out its contents. His jaw dropped as soon as his eyes registered what was in front of him.

On the front page, I had drawn a lad - who looked a lot like Dean - enjoying his first driving lesson a little too much, terrifying his balding instructor. Inside, the paper car popped out as if, I hoped, it was coming off the road. Dean laughed heartily at that.

'I'll try not to cause too much devastation today,' he chuckled. 'But wow, Loz, this is brilliant! You're a star, mate - thanks, again!'

He held the card delicately between his fingers and studied my design. It might have been a priceless masterpiece for all the care he took.

I felt the colour in my cheeks rise. 'It's…just a little something.'

'This is more than just a *little something.*' He grimaced slightly. 'I think whatever happens today, *this* will outshine any of it by far. You could seriously make a profession out of this. You've got real talent!'

His eyes glimmered and my own began to sting. His genuine praise was touching a nerve, so I decided to change the subject.

'S-so what are your plans for today?'

'Well,…first of all, to get over this hangover!' he laughed.

I jolted up out of my seat. 'Oh, God! I'm sorry, you're right, I shouldn't have disturbed you so early.' I quickly gathered up the discarded wrapping paper around us and moved to put the chair back against the far wall. How selfishly inconsiderate I was, waking him up at such a time on his own birthday for no real reason other than to hear him sing my praises over my gifts!

'No, no!' He reached out to grab my arms, stopping me from my tidying. 'It's okay. Stay, please.'

I looked down at him, realising too late that he had, once again, unleashed his eye-power on me. I fluttered a little as I spoke, 'If you're sure I'm not being a pain…'

'Nah…No more than usual.' He grinned wickedly. 'Anyway, I

guess I really shouldn't sleep away the day. I only get one birthday a year.'

Out of the corner of my eye, I noticed again the book on his bedside table.

'What are you reading, there?' I asked as I went to pick it up. The image on the cover intrigued me; it looked like a flying saucer.

'Ah, erm, it's nothing...' Dean answered nervously, springing quickly to seize it from out of my reach. But I beat him to it.

I picked it up and read the shiny, purple embossed words out loud, '"Is There Anybody Out There?"'

'It's nothing,' he said again. I looked back at him to see him twiddling with the sheets. His cheeks had gone a little rosy, too. I had never seen him this agitated before; It was quite endearing.

I repressed a smile. 'This is a book on alien life forms, isn't it?' I was greatly amused, as well as surprised.

'Err...yeah, maybe.' He shrugged. 'You think it's silly, I know.'

I opened the first page to read the in-cover blurb and was astonished to find that there was also a library ticket glued inside.

I tittered. 'I never knew.'

'Never knew what?'

'That you were such a geek at heart!' I joked, snapping the book closed and putting it back down. It was kind of a relief, actually, to know that there was so much more depth to this young man than what I already knew, and it just made me love him all the more.

He gave me a playful kick, finding it hard to keep from smiling, himself.

'No, really,' I said, thinking for a moment for the right words, 'it's, err, "cute."'

He smirked. 'Shut-up!'

I slid myself onto the edge of his bed and picked up the ball of scrunched up wrapping paper, playing with it idly between my fingers. 'So. You have fun last night, then?'

'It was just a little gathering round Randy's. We played a lot of silly party games. Most of which involved drinking vast quantities of alcohol.'

'Of course.'

'Jammy was a complete knob-head, though!' He scowled.

'Oh?' No surprise there.

'Yeah…Well, you know Randy's girlfriend…?'

Dean had mentioned her to me before. Her name was Celeste, and, at only 20, she had already made Randy an official toy-boy. She was also an ex-stripper; I didn't know where at, though. As far as I was concerned, most of the people of Suffolk had no idea what a strip club was. I nodded for Dean to continue with the story.

'Well, by the time Jammy had arrived, he was already quite pissed. He'd never met Celeste before and couldn't get over the idea that she used to be a stripper. He wanted to know why she'd bothered to give it up at all, since the pay's supposed to be so great.

'She said that she only needed the money in the first place, because she lives away from home and, as well as funding college on the side, she needed rent money. But in the end, after a load of dangerous encounters with stalkers, she decided it wasn't worth it and packed it up.

'Jammy wouldn't drop the subject, though. He contradicted himself and said that he, personally, wouldn't give "those" girls the time of day, let alone his hard earned cash, saying that they were all thieves and STI-ridden skanks, anyway.'

I gasped. Though the viciousness of his comments wasn't all that out of character, I was surprised that Jammy had had the balls to say it in front of a group of friends. And especially to one of their girlfriends!

'What did Randy have to say to that?'

'He was outside having a ciggy at the time, so missed it all. In any case, he was just as drunk as Jammy. We still all told Jammy off for it, though. Not that Celeste wasn't more than capable of holding her own against him, mind.'

'What did she do?' I leant in. This was fun gossip!

His lips curled up slightly. 'She threw her drink in his face and told him to go fuck himself.'

I couldn't not laugh. 'God, how I wish I could have seen that!… Or done the honours!'

'Jammy left shortly after that. You were right, he really is such an arsehole!'

I was quick to point out that Jammy's range of arsehole-ness had always been limitless.

'Why you even bother with him is beyond me,' I sighed.

'I have to put up with him. He kinda comes as a package deal with the rest of them.'

'Which also baffles me! You've mentioned before how their superficial banter is beginning to annoy you,' I said exasperatedly.

'Hey, I've got to fit in somewhere…'

'You would always fit in with me and the guys,'

'Wrong. I'd fit in with just you. I don't think your friends like me all that much.'

'They like you…well enough.' I was a terrible liar.

'Ha! I knew it!' he chuckled.

'Alright, so neither one of us gets on with the other's friends. That's now a given.'

There was a short pause

'I kinda like it this way, though, you know,' he said thoughtfully.

'You do?' Though I was secretly in avid agreement and sitting on tenterhooks waiting for his next thoughts. I was in danger of ripping the paper in my hands to shreds in my anticipation.

'Yeah, I do,' he said, his luminous eyes on me, shining so brilliantly that I had to catch my breath. 'I just feel like I can be more like my real self around you than I can when I'm with the others.

'I mean, with them it's all football this, cars that, getting pissed this, fit birds that. And I don't mind sometimes, but it gets so trivial. I just feel like I can shake a lot of that off when I'm around you. No faking it.'

I considered this, then grinned broadly. 'I think I'm in danger of being overly flattered.'

He laughed a little at that. Then, when he stopped, he really stared at me. I dropped my expression, and turned away and pinked.

'You know, when you smile, you get a tiny, little dimple on the side of your left cheek,' he said nonchalantly.

The statement stunned and confused me a little. 'Really? I hadn't noticed.' I really hadn't, but I would be sure to check.

'It's just something I've observed.'

I put a hand to my face self-consciously. I wasn't sure how to take this. 'Is it a good thing?'

He chuckled softly. 'Why would it be a bad thing?'

'I dunno. I guess I'm just not used to compliments.'

What did all this mean coming from him?

I wanted to reciprocate in some way, to even the score, but I knew that whatever I said would only come across as a borderline crazy stalker observation. I mean, how could I possibly tell him that I thought the little furrow he got between his eyes whenever he knitted his brows was painfully adorable? How could I tell him that I had memorised the exact positions of all three moles on the back of his right hand? How could I tell him that I dreamt about running my fingers over the faded birthmark that was artistically placed at the tip of his right elbow? And how could I even possibly think of telling him that every night I dreamt about feeling his hard body up against mine and...

'What are you thinking?' he asked, mercifully interrupting my train of thought.

I answered dazedly, 'I was thinking about what else to say to that.'

'You don't have to say anything.'

But I thought for a moment longer, anyway.

'I like your hair.' It was a bit of a lame response, but I decided it was all I could come up with without making myself glaringly obvious. 'In that it does things mine doesn't...Mine's all kinda fluffy and weird.'

I was starting to sweat now, I realised. I must have sounded like an utter moron.

Dean snickered. 'You make me laugh, Laurence Price.'

I tried to relax a little. 'Not at me, I hope.'

'Not always.' He winked.

We both laughed.

'And another thing - your laugh!'

'Oh, God!' I hid my face in shame. 'That bad, is it? I must sound like Goofy on helium!'

'Yeah, but it's funny!' His face was vastly amused.

'I bet it'll grate on you after a while...Anyway, what's with all the scrutiny?'

'What?'

'What's suddenly so interesting about me?'

He sniggered. 'You've always been pretty interesting, Loz.'

I grimaced. 'But what *is* so interesting?'

I noticed I was beginning to sound desperate, now. What I really wanted to say was how could *I* possibly interest *him*. I honestly didn't see how I could be worth his time and attention.

Dean just eyed me intently. He looked like he was about to say something else, but then seemed to backtrack. 'I don't know. But it's something.' He smiled weakly.

My heart skipped a beat as he then threw back the covers and rose out of bed. My eyes wondered mischievously after him as he walked over to the door - where his dressing gown hung from the hook - wearing only a holey top and a pair of boxers. The wrapping paper rustled violently within my grasp and I quickly turned my head away, suppressing the natural urge that growled within me.

I couldn't help but think about what I had seen. I thought about those strong legs and the light, downy hairs that coated them. I was afraid my eyes would be drawn back to him. It was hard work to restrain myself.

'It's okay, it's not like I'm naked,' he chortled. He must have thought I was embarrassed by the sight. 'There. Decent enough for you?'

I didn't answer, but I dared myself to look over, anyway, and he was now safely wrapped in his dressing gown. Thankfully, he didn't seem to have any idea how perilously close he had come to being pounced on!

'Oh, by the way...' he started. 'A little last minute plan concocted last night, but Cyndi Langham wants to host another party for me tonight. She says her parents needed to get out of town at short notice and so now she's got the house to herself.'

'Oh?...' Did this have any relevance for me?

'And, well, I was wondering if you wanted to come.'

His expression was unreadable as he waited for my response. I really wasn't sure about it, though. 'Will *all* your friends be there?' I asked hesitantly.

He came and sat back down next to me on the unmade bed. 'Yeah...And look, I know you don't like most of them--'

Meaning, of course, *all* of them - *especially* Jammy!

'--but it *is* my birthday, after all...' He pleaded at me with his striking eyes and best smile. He must have sensed that would win me over, hands down.

'Oh, alright,' I sighed, fighting back a grin. 'I'll come, but *only* because it's your birthday.'

'Great!' He bounced. He seemed genuinely excited, now. 'And don't worry, I promise not to use that excuse again for a whole year!'

I felt a multitude of emotions then. He planned on still knowing me in a year?

'Right. Well, I'm gonna have to start getting ready now, so...'

I was momentarily lost in a heavenly daydream of possibilities at that moment and wasn't really paying much attention. '...Huh?'

'So...' he said more forcibly, hinting at the door with a tilt of his head.

'Oh, right, sure. Yeah, no worries, I'll get out of your hair,' I blundered in realisation, scurrying out the room with the thoroughly screwed up wrapping paper.

The rest of the day went by pretty smoothly. We did the whole present giving scene again downstairs with the families later that morning, as well as had the cake for breakfast (of which Dean loved, his glowing face saying it all, and I was inwardly very smug).

Bonnie's own gift to her son was ten weeks worth of driving lessons all prepaid for. However, this was not without hinting that he would need to start paying for further ones himself. I caught him scowling behind his mother's back. He would need to job hunt soon.

That evening, at around 8:00pm, and both dressed in our smart-casual bests, Dean and I set off for Cyndi's place.

The air was crisp, and on the way, Dean filled me in on his first lesson from earlier that afternoon, boasting how he was so obviously a born-natural driver. He then listed for me some of the cars he hoped to someday own. A part of me died on hearing this; he was so definitely straight.

'You can start giving me lifts to school, then,' I half-laughed, trying to mask my suffering.

'For a small fee, sure,' he joked, nudging me.

I just smiled absentmindedly.

'Are you okay, Loz?'

I forced myself to smile more sincerely. 'Yeah, no, I'm fine. Honest. I'm just glad you've had a good day, that's all.'

But just like everyone else, he must have thought he could see right through me.

'Please don't worry about tonight, mate. I really appreciate your coming,' he said genuinely, stopping me.

'...Well, thanks for inviting me.' My tone was emotionless.

The corners of his mouth twitched upwards. 'At least *try* to enjoy it, eh?'

I tried to look appalled at his insinuation, but I knew I had failed. 'I will *try*,' I said in defeat. 'Lucky lad, you are, though - two parties!'

'I know! Last night was meant to be it, really. Some of my friends in the upper sixth have got bar or restaurant jobs on weekend nights, see. But Cyndi was adamant that she'd rustle up something else for me tonight on my *actual* birthday.'

I stared ahead while he talked, and as we carried on walking through the darkened streets, I decided then to just come out with it.

'You know she fancies you, right?'

This seemed to take him by surprise. '*What?*'

'Cyndi. You can't tell me you don't already know!'

'No, I don't.' He sounded serious as he turned his burning eyes on me. The moonlight reflected off of them so mystically, though, that it inadvertently softened his manner.

'She follows you around like a shadow, Dean, and she dotes on you like a puppy! Just look at what she's thrown together at the last minute for you!' I said in exasperation.

The cogs in his head seemed to be turning as he absorbed my information.

'Hmm.'

'You see?'

He puffed his cheeks out and threw his hands around his head, not knowing what else to do with them. 'O-kay...' he said after a while.

'Of course, none of this would matter if you really liked her.' I paused, looking closely for any sign of intent in the idea. There was none, and his subsequent reaction pleased me to no end.

'No! God, no! Not like *that*!' he said disgustedly.

'Alright, but maybe you need to tell her that before she has anymore wild misconceptions about the two of you.'

My argument was furthermore justified as we rounded the bend towards Cyndi's house.

It was an eyesore; there was certainly no danger of a party decoration shortage. The outside was almost covered from the roof to the ground with paper lanterns, bunched balloons and multicoloured fairy lights. I shuddered to think how she managed to adorn parts of the house without needing a hazardously long ladder!

We could hear Cyndi's trendy play list pulsating away as we walked up the long, tidily gravelled driveway. Cars were parked in every available space; from right up close to the house, to along the gate, and even up on the grass verge of the green opposite the large, elegant, Georgian-style country home.

There seemed to be a large amount of chatter emanating from within, as well. Thank goodness for her nearest neighbours that they at least lived a few yards up the road.

'Oh, Lord!' Dean groaned, eyeing the place over.

'Aw, at least *try* to have fun, eh?' I teased, as I banged the knocker on the overly generous-sized front door.

CHAPTER 13.

We weren't waiting long before the door was thrown open, revealing a very dressy and excitable Cyndi Langham.

'Yay, everyone! The birthday boy's here!' she squealed over the crowd behind her in the large and alarmingly bright hallway. 'Ooh, and you brought Loz, too!'

I got the distinct feeling that the other guests neither knew or really gave a damn about me *or* Dean, in all honesty. They seemed to pay little, if any, interest in our arrival.

'Hey, Cynd!' Dean gave a little wave. He looked nervous, now, seeing the mass of people that steadily encroached upon us. I saw in his eyes that Cyndi's doting infatuation with him was, at last, screamingly evident. I just smiled politely as we were let in.

'Want any snacks, guys? They're in the kitchen through here,' she said, pointing over her shoulder, armed with a coke-and-something held daintily between her fingers. She led us around the sea of - I assumed - sixth formers, who were bopping away and chatting intermittently above the music.

You could tell Cyndi had really gone all out tonight; her appearance alone was enough to put every other girl here to shame. I was just glad, and still a little bowled over by the fact, that her charm and beauty, apparently, held absolutely no interest for Dean whatsoever.

As we went through, he nodded and smiled obligingly to random people he did recognise, but I got the impression that not even he was quite expecting *this* kind of turn out.

Once in the kitchen, Cyndi motioned us towards the breakfast table - posing as a makeshift buffet and drinks table - and then made to leave us to it.

'You two just help yourselves. I'll go see if I can find the others.'

Before she could go, however, Dean quickly grabbed her hand and pulled her to one side. 'Whoa, whoa, Cynd! I thought you said this was just going to be a *small* gathering,' he said in hushed speech, but not so quietly that I couldn't hear him.

'This *is* small, babe. Don't you like it?' she sounded hurt, but her china doll-like face remained impassive.

I looked around, taking in my surroundings. The inside of the house was worse than the outside; it was like looking at the aftermath of a balloon factory explosion - helium-filled decorations *everywhere*! Paper chains festooned the walls, and Dixie cups and used drinks bottles of the fizzy, soft and alcoholic kind littered every available surface. Cyndi was deliberately trying to prove a point by all of this, and I felt satisfied in the knowledge that it had, ironically, had the reverse affect.

'It's great, Cynd,' I lied, answering for Dean.

'Thanks, hon.' She beamed at me. I was glad she couldn't see through me like most people could.

'Yeah, it's nice, Cynd, but I don't even know most of these people,' Dean said shortly.

Her face grew a little annoyed by his response. 'Oh, so I invited a few extra people--'

'*A few*?!' he exclaimed.

'Yes, *a few*! Hell, it's my house, Dean! Whether it's your birthday or not, I can invite whoever I bloody well want into my own home!' she spat.

I was knocked for six. I had never known Cyndi to snap before.

'Happy Birthday, Dean!' she sniffed, dejected. And with that, she stormed off, presumably in search of friends for a shoulder to bitch to.

'That wasn't very grateful,' I admonished him once she had gone, while helping myself to a paper plate and a handful of party-sized sausage rolls.

He sighed heavily, copying me. 'I know, I know.'

'You do see what I mean, though?' I pressed.

'Definitely! But, what am I gonna do?'

'Well, there doesn't seem to be a lot you can do tonight,' I said honestly. 'Just enjoy what she's done here, but perhaps keep a low profile with her for a while.'

I amazed myself with how insightful I sounded. I was good at this counselling lark.

'You're right,' he breathed, looking at me with relief. 'Thanks, mate.'

'Hey, that's what I'm here for.'

We moved round the buffet table and grabbed a few napkins.

'You're sixteen already, aren't you?' he asked suddenly.

I looked at him. 'Erm, yeah. Since September 2nd , remember?' I was sure I had told him that before.

It had been a fairly low-key affair, my birthday - only a few days before I had met Dean for the first time. Dad had done a barbeque for me and the guys, but that had been it. I didn't like people making a fuss over me; it always made me feel uncomfortable, being the centre of attention.

'I still can't believe that.' He smiled a small, musing smile. 'You seem to have more sense for your age than half the kids here, I'm sure, and they must all be at least two years older than you!'

Once again, I could feel my cheeks colour fiercely at his words.

'Do you want a drink? I'm gagging for a beer,' he announced.

'Err, sure. A vodka and lemonade would be great, thanks,' I assented, trying to hide my beetroot-tinted face.

As he went to pour them out, I held onto his plate. We then decided to go and explore Cyndi's mansion.

Both hands now full, I hadn't really thought about how I was actually going to eat my food, so I quickly downed my drink, winced, then stuffed my face with crisps to get rid of the aftertaste. Though I was gradually becoming accustomed to alcohol, I still only ever felt the need for it in social situations; it loosened me up a bit.

As we walked back out into the buzzing hallway, I noticed little Bern sitting huddled on the upstairs' step, peeping through the banister at what was going on down below. He must have been under strict instruction not to interfere with the party. If I knew Bern, though, it wasn't like him to comply so dutifully to such a request. My guess was that Cyndi had blackmailed him with something in order to a) keep him out of the way, and b) make sure he didn't mention any of this to the parents.

He scowled when he saw me, pouting like a small child - he looked like one compared to everyone else here. I knew exactly what he was thinking, too: why was I allowed here when I was only a year older than him? I suppose at our age, though, every year made a difference to levels of maturity. I was, however, glad that, at least according to Dean, I could easily pass off as a member of this more senior club.

'Do you think Cyndi's got the *whole* of sixth form here?' Dean asked, snapping my attention away from the forlorn-looking tenth year.

'Looks like it, doesn't it.'

We managed to find an impossibly empty spot in the corner of the long hallway, where we stood watching out over the crowd. I felt like an on-looking naturalist on a documentary show, observing and analysing people's social behavioural patterns.

'Not that there's a shortage of guests or anything, but who else were you expecting to be here?' I said, noticing him scanning the faces around us.

'Well, Harry for one; Jammy, too; and a couple of my upper sixth mates from P.E. But I can't even see *them*! I swear, half these people don't even go to Audley!'

'Hey, Dean!' someone called from behind me.

I whipped round to find a podgy lad in khaki trousers and a baggy, beer-stained, white shirt squeezing his way through the mob, his arms waving madly in the air for attention. Dean looked immensely relieved.

'That's Pete Tubbs - or just *Tubbs*,' he said to me, seeing my bemused expression. An apt name, I thought cruelly.

'Deano, how are you?' Tubbs shouted out over the background noise. He made his way over and shook Dean firmly by the hand. His face was dripping with sweat and I cringed involuntarily at the sight of him. Had he been in better shape, he might otherwise have looked okay, but as it was, he had a body as round as a beach ball and, subsequently, a hideously swollen-looking face. You could barely make out his more detailed features - they were all swallowed up by the rolls of fat. I scolded myself for my prejudice.

'I'm fine, dude. You?' Dean said, happy to finally see someone else he properly knew and liked.

'Cool, cool. And listen, Happy Birthday!'

'Cheers, mate.' He smiled appreciatively. 'You enjoying the party?'

'Ah, yeah, it's wicked!' Tubbs answered animatedly - he certainly looked like he was having a good time.

Tubbs' eyes then switched to me, assessing me, and suddenly Dean seemed to remember I was there.

'Oh, shit! Sorry, Tubbs. This is Loz - he's a friend of mine.'

"Friend"…Great.

'Oh? I've not seen you around the sixth form,' said Tubbs, glaring superiorly at me.

'Oh, I'm not in the sixth form yet,' I said.

'I see.'

And that was all I got before he turned back to Dean.

Dean's friends had a habit of looking over me like that, and it was really beginning to annoy me. It was as if they could sense how insignificant I was, even if he couldn't.

'I take it you know most of these people?' Dean asked, motioning his head towards the horde of party goers before us.

'Of course! I'm the life and soul here, Deany-ma-boy!' he said, as if that were obvious. I couldn't tell whether or not that was just delusion on his part, though. 'Don't worry, I'll hook you up, mate. Just come with me.'

Before I had even had time to register that Dean was gone, he was already halfway across the hall, being forcibly dragged away by the arm by his eager friend. I was now alone.

'Bugger!' I hissed irritably through gritted teeth. This was the last thing I needed!

I made a point of following after them, but I had already lost them before I could even work out which direction they had gone in.

I noticed two doors to adjoining rooms had been opened, and people flowed in and out. But, though they did, the hallway was, if possible, becoming even more unbearably cramped. So much so, that I was fast becoming wedged between the wall of people in front of me and the concrete one I stood in front of.

With my back now pressed firmly against the wall, I slid round the room until I reached the kitchen; it was the only other room in this house that I had properly explored, and hoped - maybe vainly - that Dean had been led back there.

He hadn't.

Ugh, I knew this party was a bad idea!…Maybe not necessarily to this degree, but a bad one, nonetheless!

I decided to stay put. I knew I would only get very lost if I tried to find Dean on my own. I was fairly confident in thinking that he would come looking for me soon, anyhow.

I watched idly by as people passed me, beverage and snacks in hand, having a great time, while I just waited, bored.

I glumly went and poured myself another drink…Then another… And then another. Pretty soon, I was on my fifth, and was beginning to feel increasingly pissed off, as well as a bit pissed.

Having now been sat alone on a stool to the side of the buffet for almost forty-five minutes, and fuelled by newfound drunken confidence, I decided I was at last feeling brave enough to search the rest of the house from top to bottom for Dean. If he wasn't coming to find me, then I would go and find him, instead, and demand that we go home!

As I rose unstably to my feet, I mixed myself a final drink for the road, and then contemplated which room off of the large family kitchen I would explore first.

The house was getting so full, people were even spilling outside. This was definitely saying something, because it was, indeed, a big house! I pitied Cyndi for all the cleaning she would no doubt be doing in the morning. But then, knowing her luck, she probably had an army of servants for that kind of stuff - the lucky cow!

Just as I planned to dive into what I thought looked like it could be the dining room, I noticed Jammy out of the corner of my eye. Though I guessed he would be here, I had secretly wished he wouldn't be. When we had arrived earlier, I rather hoped that, since there were so many people here, the chances of me actually bumping into him would be slim. It was, of course, typical that he would find me while I was on my own, defenceless!

He was coming in from outside via the big French double doors that lead into the kitchen, a box of cigarettes in one hand and a drink in the other. Luckily, it looked like he hadn't seen me, yet.

Seeking the nearest sanctuary, I hurriedly ducked behind the kitchen cum buffet table.

It was fortunate that the tablecloth was long, because if I wanted to, I might even have got away with hiding *under* the table. But, realising that I had already attracted a few head turns for my sudden peculiar behaviour, I decided I probably shouldn't go quite that far.

I poked my head over the edge to see if he was gone, only to find him looking directly me…as well as many others.

'Pricey?' his horribly familiar voice called. I could hear the funeral march playing away in the back of my mind. He started cackling to himself at the sight of me. 'You're here?'

'I-I was invited,' I said petulantly.

He came over and towered over me. I forgot I was still kneeling.

'And on the floor?' he asked. This seemed to highly amuse him.

'I, err…just dropped my, my…drink! Yes! I dropped my drink.'

It was only then that I noticed my drink was actually sitting safely on the table at eyelevel with my hand wrapped protectively around it. Crap! Well, I did say I was a bad liar, didn't I?

'Really?' He raised one eyebrow skeptically and glanced at the half-full cup in my grasp. I quickly let go of it and moved my hand away.

'Uh-huh,' I mumbled, embarrassed, and getting up to dust down my trousers.

''Kay, whatever.' He sneered, leering at me. I didn't like the gleam in his eyes; they were dark and untrustworthy. I wished he would go.

'Can I help you?' I asked aggressively.

He grimaced at my tone. 'I'm getting a drink, *actually*. This *is* the food and drinks table, isn't it?'

I kept quiet at that. The other onlookers were now, thankfully, minding their own business.

'You want another one? Since you "dropped" your last one and all,' he said scornfully.

I did fancy another drink, I just didn't need *him* to get it for me.

'No, that's okay I--'

But he had already gone over to do it, anyway.

'Vodka and coke alright?' he asked.

I eyed him curiously. I guessed it couldn't do me any harm. There were too many people around for Jammy to start something. None of his back-up crew seemed to be here, either. And anyway, he was being uncharacteristically nice for a change; I might as well roll with it while it lasted.

'Sure. Thanks.'

I went and sat back down on my stool, looked about distractedly and waited for my drink.

'Here,' he said, coming over and handing me the fizzing cup.

He stood for a few moments, sipping at his drink and watching me nurse my own.

'Anything else?' I demanded. This was as far as my cordiality would allow. I knew I was being rude, but nice or not, going on our history together, Jammy Jobson hardly deserved any respect from me!

'*Jeez*! Crabby tonight, aren't we?!' He scowled.

'Only around you.'

He bent down and leant in close to me so that I could smell his smoky, boozy breath.

'And why's that, Pricey?'

'You know why.' I glared back at him.

'Hmm.' He smiled mockingly, his all-seeing eyes examining my face. Then he straightened back up, ruffled my hair patronisingly and stalked off. 'Seeya later, Pricey.'

I stared after him and self-consciously rearranged my hair. God, how I hated that boy!

But still, in spite of having none of his posse to show off to, for Jammy, that was a remarkably easy meeting. I had expected him to at least find someway of making a show of me, to humiliate me in front of everyone, like he usually did. But he hadn't; he hadn't stuck around long enough for any of that. Maybe I had just got him on one of his very seldom "nice" days.

Momentarily abandoning my plans to search for Dean, I thought about this. In fact, I thought about a lot of things, though not all of them making much sense. Faces started coming in and out of focus, and I suddenly felt quite weak and drowsy. I must have been more drunk than I thought. Staying sat where I was, was becoming a much more attractive idea than going traipsing around a two storey mansion. Maybe if I just shut my eyes for a second, too...

❧

Dean had found himself in the dining room, where the dining room table was being used as a second, more generously stocked buffet / drinks table.

He was in the middle of a conversation with a girl he had never met before, but whom Tubbs had introduced him to. Her name was Sarah Smart, she was in the upper sixth, and she was definitely showing an overly keen interest in him. Dean just wanted to get away.

He noticed Tubbs in the corner, cracking a joke with a circle of admirers. He was The Funny Guy and everyone loved him; his enthusiasm for things was contagious.

But Dean was done, now. This party was turning out to be a real disappointment. He had clearly upset Cyndi, who he hadn't seen again since he had arrived; he hadn't seen any of his real mates, bar Tubbs, for all the people that were here; it was *his* birthday, and hardly anyone here even knew who he was; and to top it off, he had lost Loz in thick of it all. Dean felt especially guilty about that part, having literally bribed his closest ally to come with him - even though Loz hadn't initially wanted to - and now he had gone and lost him!

Dean had been in the room for almost an hour, now, and in that time, he had been passed from group to group like a parcel. Some of the people were okay, but he couldn't really sense any lasting friendships blossoming. Most of them would probably become acquaintances at best.

Finally deciding enough was enough, Dean prised himself away from Sarah's adoring advances, and carefully made his way around the obstacle course of people in order to reach Tubbs.

'And then he says to the other guy--Oh! Hey, Dean! I was just in the middle of--'

'Tubbs, I'm gonna go find Loz, okay?' Dean said, patting his friend on the shoulder and moving off, not waiting for a response.

It took him almost five minutes to navigate his way out of the absurdly overcrowded room. As he pushed through, he noticed the rather disgruntled-looking Jo Reiner, who was alone and standing hidden away under an alcove, sipping away at her drinks cup and gazing moodily at the people around her. Dean just ignored her. She was a strange one, that Jo Reiner, and he had always suspected that she particularly didn't like him, for whatever reason.

Once he had made it back to the kitchen in one piece - where things were only marginally less congested, but still clear enough for him to, at last, see Loz tucked away to the far side - Dean breathed a sigh of relief; Loz hadn't got far. But then when Dean looked a little closer at him, his heart gave an almighty thud.

His head slumped and a drink held precariously within his weakened clasp, something was definitely not right with Loz.

Everything then went quiet for Dean. All he could see was Loz, all he could hear was his own steadily accelerating heartbeat, and all he could feel was a deepening sense of distress. Loz's wellbeing was suddenly more important to him than anything he had ever cared about before.

He barged past people, not caring who he knocked, and paid no attention to their indignant protests. He rushed to Loz's side, grabbed the drink off of him and tilted his head upwards by the chin. Loz groaned. At least he was alive, Dean thought mercifully, the knot in his stomach loosening only very slightly.

'Loz! Loz, it's Dean! Are you okay, mate?' he cried fretfully. He gently patted Loz's unusually pale cheeks to generate more consciousness. It worked. His once firmly shut eyes forced themselves open half a fraction, and his lips pressed into a small smile in recognition.

'Hi, Dean,' he said feebly.

Dean answered with a wide grin of his own. 'Hey, you! Are you okay? You don't look so hot.'

'Thanks,' Loz replied lazily.

'What's wrong?'

'I'm not feeling too well,' he mumbled.

'Yeah, I gathered that. Was it something you ate? Did you drink too much?'

It seemed to take Loz a few moments to string the next sentence together in his head.

'I was...fine a minute ago,...and then Jammy came, and then he...'

Dean's guts squeezed uncomfortably, and immeasurable anger boiled up inside of him. Jammy? What had *he* done?

'Loz, you have to tell me. What did Jammy do?'

Loz looked confused at the seriousness of Dean's tone. 'He made me a...a drink.'

The hairs stood up on the nape of Dean's neck. This was not normal drunkenness Loz was experiencing, and it didn't take a genius to see that something was seriously wrong with the way he was at the moment. Had Jammy *spiked* Loz?

'Shit, Loz! We've gotta get you to a hospital!'

'A hosp--why?' he squeaked. He was still struggling to keep his head elevated on his own.

'Because I think you've been drugged, mate,' Dean said darkly. But this didn't seem to register with the incoherent Loz. It didn't make much sense to Dean, either. Why *would* Jammy do something like that?

In spite of this being a very awkward, and potentially life threatening, scene, barely anyone had taken a blind bit of notice at what was going on. The room was too busy, too noisy, the people too drunk to care. Dean couldn't worry about them, though. As soon as the paramedics got here, they would all know then that something was up.

Dean felt around in his pockets for his mobile. 'Damn it!' he growled, slapping his palm to his forehead. The one time he actually forgot his phone! He looked about him in an attempt to locate Cyndi's house phone, but to no avail.

'Dean?...I think...I think I'm gonna be sick,' Loz whimpered, trying to get up.

'Shit, okay!' Dean thought about this. Loz really needed medical attention, but maybe being sick would help to empty his system. 'Right, this way, then,' he said decisively.

Dean pulled Loz's arm over his shoulder and almost carried him through to the utility room where the toilet was situated just off of it.

Still no-one paid any attention to them as they stumbled their way past. In their eyes, they were probably just two pissed mates larking about.

Leaving Loz to his own devices in the toilet, Dean put an ear to the door and was pleased to hear that he was, indeed, throwing up. The less there was in him, the better. Maybe the drowsiness would wear off soon, as well.

'Loz, stay put for a sec, okay? I'm just going to find a phone. I'll be back soon,' he called. There was a murmured response, but Dean didn't have time to clarify. Loz would probably be in there for a while, anyway.

Dean headed back into the main part of the house, and, finding the first person he could, asked to borrow a phone. He then dialled for the emergency services.

'Bollocks! No signal,' he groaned. This could not be happening! 'Do you mind, mate, if I take this outside? It *is* an emergency.'

The guy whose phone he had borrowed didn't seem to like that idea. But while Dean understood that the guy was reluctant to hand his phone over to a complete stranger, he couldn't waste even more time trying to convince him.

'Look, you can follow me outside if you want,' he said, exasperated.

The guy eventually agreed, and Dean hurried with him back out to the utility room to the back door. Just as they passed through, however, Dean noticed that the toilet door was wide open and there was no Loz in sight.

CHAPTER 14.

I felt strange.

Someone was tugging at me by the arm and I was walking. The motion part did *not* make me feel good. It also didn't help my vision much, blurring it even more as I watched the, already distorted, faces around me disappear into nothingness.

I guessed I must have been outside, because there was suddenly less light and it was very cold. My arms were bare to the elements; had I come without a jacket?

I was led onto something squishy; it might have been grass. I heard a creak and a gentle bang, of which sounded like the opening and closing of a gate. I then felt and heard the crunch of gravel beneath me. Where was I going?

Everything had happened so quickly. One minute I was being sick in the toilet, and then, during a breather, the door had been opened and someone - or something - had reached in and yanked me out. I hadn't had the time or mental capacity to really worry about who or what it was, though; I was still having trouble trying to focus on remembering where I was now! I was pretty sure Dean was supposed to be around here somewhere, too. Maybe it was him who was dragging me. Maybe he was just walking me home. Although I felt he was being unusually rough with me, I decided that, in the end, I was simply far too dopey to care either way. All this thinking was exhausting…

I might have fallen asleep on my feet, because when I next tried to force open my heavy eyelids, I was nowhere I recognised. It was almost black, and, from what I could tell, there was only dark wall around me.

'Dean, where are we?' I croaked. For the first time since the onset of all this sudden weirdness, I was beginning to grow anxious - a sign of alertness.

'I'm not Dean,' came a voice.

I gulped. No, he certainly was not!

I began to shiver, panic stricken. Tired or not, that voice would be enough to scare even Sleeping Beauty out from her subconscious!

'Jammy?' my own voice quivered.

'That's right,' he answered icily.

I heard the soft crackle of the ground as he stepped closer to me. My body froze. I was terrified. In crowded situations I could handle him, but alone, I had no chance.

'Wha-what's going on?' I managed, adrenaline pumping away. But despite finally feeling very awake now, my legs had turned into jelly. There was no-way I could run.

'Nothing's really going on, Pricey. I just felt that you and I should maybe have a little chat, that's all,' Jammy said, eerily calm.

'Why?' Something didn't fit. He had actively gone out of his way to get me on my own!

'We don't do it enough, do we?'

'We don't like each other,' I said wryly.

'Well, I can't really be blamed for that, now, can I? I mean, more often that not, that's your fault.'

'*What? You're* the one with the problem with *me!*' I cried out. How could he be so arrogant?!

'Ah, see, there you go again. If you're not careful, you might end up really pissing me off - like you do so well,' he said frankly.

'You're mad!'

'No, you *make* me mad!' he snarled.

I flinched. The sound of his voice was now disturbingly close. He could only be inches away from me.

'But how?' I was genuinely at a loss with this one. As far I was aware, it was always *him* who provoked *me*.

Suddenly, with a rush of air, and in one swift movement, his hands were on my shirt, and I was lifted up off the ground from where I stood and thrown.

My head bumped hard against the brick of the wall, but I

didn't fall, as he kept me pinned there. My eyes had slowly grown accustomed to the dark, and up close, I could now see Jammy's pallid face in the low moonlight - he was menacing.

'What the hell are you doing?!' I cried through the pain. 'Get off me!'

He did not answer, but glowered back at me. He seemed to be contemplating something.

'Just *leave* me alone! What have I *ever* done to you?' I choked.

'You wanna know what you've done to me, Pricey?' he taunted. His eyes were growing increasingly threatening, and his grip on my shirt tightened. 'You *exist*! That's what you've done to me, Pricey! That's *why* you piss me off so much!' he hissed.

I was slightly confused at his response, but was now also too scared for my life. I was at the hands of a madman in, what was, an empty alleyway in the backend of nowhere, and almost certainly there would be no-one close by in this tumbleweed village to save me. Whatever was in store for me, Jammy had planned it perfectly.

'What exactly am I supposed to say to that?' I breathed unevenly, petrified and mentally bracing myself for what I thought was the inevitable.

There was a chilling pause, interrupted only by panting.

'Nothing,' he eventually whispered, as if in a trance.

He continued staring at me intensely. If he was going to kill me, I rather hoped he would at least spare me the torture of enduring his mind games. This was unmistakably psychotic behaviour!

'I hate you, you know that?!' he spat. 'I hate you more than anything in the world! It's because of you that my life makes no sense, that everything is so fucked up!'

'What the hell are you talking about?!'

What was it about me that made him hate me? He had no real reason to; in all the years he had bullied me – since the start of high school - I had thought exactly that.

But then, feeling his lips fiercely pressed against mine, I got my answer.

A kiss; a kiss that kept on going, and each one that followed was as if it would be his last. It might even have been nice had he not been a complete whack-job and wasn't squashing my head into the wall. I was just too stunned to move a muscle.

Once I got my senses back, however, I squirmed away from his lips' grasp. My head throbbed and spun with fear and confusion, but he grabbed my chin, turned my face back to his and moved in again even more ardently than before. His forcefulness was hurting me more, now, and I was slowly suffocating in his mouth. He was using his forearms to pin my own flailing arms and had positioned himself right up against me as I dangled, grinding vigorously in between and up my thighs. I realised, with horror, where this would lead. He was under some sort of maddening spell and I couldn't escape. He was bigger and far stronger than me, and I was doomed to suffer whatever I had coming. I wept a silent tear as I gave into his violent passions.

Then, all of a sudden, everything went into fast forward.

Jammy was prised off of me, and I gasped for air as I slid to the gravely ground, clutching myself. There was a series of yelps and grunts – signs of a struggle, followed by the unmistakably dull thud of fists meeting flesh.

'Enough! Please, stop!' I heard Jammy snivel. My saviour was clearly ripping heavily into him, and I didn't need to be told who it was.

I wanted to reach out and have my own revenge, but not only was I not physically strong enough to defend myself against a tyrant like Jammy, but my mind was still swirling. Shaking with the shock, I was surprised I might actually live to see another day. The feeling was so overwhelming, that I spiralled into darkness.

CHAPTER 15.

The next thingI knew, I was lying on the ground, looking up at the silhouette of Dean's face against the backdrop of the star-spangled sky - even in the dark, I knew the shape of him too well. I figured I wasn't dead, at least.

'Oh, thank fuck you're okay!' he cried, as his hands flew to my cheeks. He sounded incredibly relieved. I guess I wasn't the only one who thought I might have died.

'Are you hurt anywhere?' he demanded.

I must have muttered something that vaguely resembled the word 'no,' because he gave me a broad, moonlit smile before helping me up to my feet. I was a bit shaky, but he steadied me.

'How did you find me?' were my first real words. I felt groggy.

'I asked around. A lot of people saw you being picked off,' he said mechanically. 'The drugs seem to have worn off, though; that's good.'

Drugs?

Then I thought I dimly remembered Dean mentioning something about that earlier, amidst the drowsiness. I shuddered at the thought of the types of abuse my body had been subjected to tonight.

'...And Jammy?'

'Gone. Don't worry, he won't be hurting you anymore,' he soothed, rubbing my tender arms. 'We'd better get going.'

It was an uncomfortable moment. Neither one of us knew what more to say. To be honest, though, I don't think either of us really wanted to say anything more about it - not just now, anyway. The less said on the matter, the less real it would hopefully feel.

As we walked back up a road, I saw Cyndi's illuminated house in the distance. Jammy hadn't taken me that far, then.

For the rest of the walk home, Dean and I kept relatively quiet. I was still feeling a little dizzy and shaken. Dean was adamant that I should see a doctor, but all I wanted to do was get home to bed - that would be the best remedy, I was sure.

I was struggling to believe what had just happened to me, and as visions of the awkwardness of the evening's events flitted across my memory, I knew there would be absolutely no-way any of this would be mentioned to anybody - not least Dad and Nana! I knew Dean's own silence meant that he, too, certainly wasn't planning on uttering a word about it. The prospect was simply too humiliating, and it would be pointless, I thought nonsensically, to worry people over something that was quickly foiled anyway. One thing was for sure, though, I had Dean to depend on. He would look out for me, whatever the cost. Tonight had proved that.

Once we were home, thankfully everyone was fast asleep. Dean led me up the stairs and we stopped outside my bedroom door.

'You gonna be alright tonight?' he asked concernedly.

'I think so.'

'Well, you know where I am if you need anything, okay?'

'Thanks,' I said quietly, touched. 'And thanks...for everything. I'm sorry about your birth--.'

'Shhh,' he put his finger to his lips, looking at me knowingly and with such compassionate eyes - eyes that sent harpoon-sized cupids' arrows souring into my heart - and then patted me affectionately on the shoulder. Though he left his hand there for a few seconds longer than was strictly necessary before moving away and heading off to his own room.

I wanted to reach out to him. No sooner had he left my side than I realised I needed him back beside me again. I felt distinctly less safe already.

I lay awake in bed for some time with horrifying flashbacks flooding back to me, going round and round my head on a seemingly endless loop.

The revelation that Jammy had secretly been repressing feelings for me all along, and was, therefore, the real reason he picked on me, was a lot to digest. It was oddly flattering, if a little too unreal.

Pretty soon, I couldn't stand listening to my own thoughts

anymore and I just needed to be with Dean - his presence seemed to make everything alright.

Without hesitation, I got out of bed and tiptoed out of my room and across the landing to his door. I knocked lightly, but entered anyway, despite knowing he was probably asleep. However, it appeared that he *had* heard me, after all. He must have been a light sleeper, either that or he was as restless as I was that night. He merely blinked at me for a couple of seconds before rising to throw a pillow to the end of his bed and lifted the duvet for me. I crept in and took in the aroma of my surroundings and his warmth, and then fell into a dreamless, deep sleep.

We topped and tailed that night, and I knew I wouldn't have traded that moment for the world.

CHAPTER 16.

This new sleeping ritual carried on for some time, while I lived in complete denial of the horrible incident.

I didn't even have to ask Dean's permission to creep into his room late each night; he just seemed to expect it, and welcomed me in each time. He seemed to understand my trauma, and realised that, for whatever reason, allowing me to share a bed with him was putting my mind at ease. This was true in many respects, but at the same time, I was also using it as an excuse for other more selfish reasons.

Some nights, I would lay awake for hours in disbelief that Dean was lying right next to me, that I was in his sheets - his sweet-smelling sheets. Sometimes, his naked leg would accidentally brush against my bare arm as he moved in his sleep, and each time my skin would prickle, my loins would ache with frustration. I had to restrain myself, but it was deliberate torture and I couldn't get enough. Often, I would be so tempted to touch him back, to stroke his masculine, toned limbs as he rested. But, sensibly, I would stop myself in time. What if he wasn't fully asleep? What if he felt me touch him? I didn't even want to think how he might react. I loved him too much to allow myself to witlessly let down my guard.

Seeing Dean pass by at school, now, was just as torturous. He would always give me a reassuringly warm smile whenever he walked past me with his mates, but I would be screaming inside. All I wanted to do was block out everyone else and pretend it was only me and him standing there. Together, alone; just so that nobody could have him in their sights but me. It made me feel so pathetic, but that's just how it was.

In the nights sometimes, if it wasn't another nightmare, my yearning torments would get to me so much that I would wake up violently - in Dean's bed, as was normal - distressed and breathless. I would want to cry out, grab him and shake him up to force him to see what he had inadvertently done to me. By which point, I was almost sympathising with Jammy! The psycho that he was, I was starting to relate to the ardency of his desires towards me.

On one of those agonising nights, Dean had obviously heard me stirring and lifted his head to see if I was okay. He didn't need to ask me, though, he knew I wasn't. And so, he clambered out from under the covers and moved down to my end of the bed. He muscled in next to me and lay on his side, staring wide-eyed at me.

'It's okay,' he whispered, patting my chest. My heart beat, synchronising with the beat of his hand. Then he stopped. He let his hand rest on my chest and did not move it. I glared hungrily into his face. The room was practically pitch black with the exception of a slither of moonlight that crept in through a gap in the curtains, illuminating our closeness.

The scene was so serene that, on impulse, and with my heart flailing wildly, I moved into him and I kissed him.

I pulled away almost as quickly as I moved in, mortified at what I had just done. But Dean hadn't even flinched, nor did he say a word. He just looked at me, so intently that I could see his eyes glisten in the limited light, and again I stared back. He began to gently massage my chest and I was instantly on fire from his touch. I sensed his curiosity matched my growing arousal as he moved his hand downwards, and further down still until he reached me.

From there, I was in ecstasy.

❧

Dean's heart pounded away like a drill against his naked breast. The very thought of what he and Loz had just done together excited him all the more.

Loz lay into him, his head resting in the nook of Dean's arm, nestled closely to his chest, so that Dean could feel his lightly inhaling and exhaling breath on his skin. Each breath tingled and sent his body quivering with desire, but he would not disturb Loz, not wanting to ruin the moment. Instead, he stared down at him, smelt the deliciously fruity fragrance of the shampoo in his hair and squeezed him to him a little tighter, enjoying the pleasing smoothness of his beautifully porcelain white skin under his touch. He didn't want to let go. He couldn't let go - not even if he *had* wanted to. He liked that Loz was here, it felt comfortable and right. And anyway, this was how Loz needed him.

No words were exchanged, and pretty soon Dean began to feel Loz's body grow limp as he drifted off into, hopefully, undisturbed sleep. Dean didn't want to go to sleep at that moment, however. He wanted to relish this peaceful moment for just a little longer, to enjoy Loz the way he was before eventually succumbing to the will of the sandman, himself.

It was very hard to see anything in the dead of night, but then he didn't need proper lighting to know Loz's every detail - they had been etched on his mind from the very moment he had laid eyes on him.

He had been immediately drawn to Loz's innocence, and the face that said it all while almost saying nothing at the same time. Something about Loz made him smile automatically every time he looked at him, or even thought about him. He had perfectly soft features; large, heart-meltingly chocolate brown eyes, and shapely, emphatic eyebrows. Dean even found Loz's hair exciting, constantly fascinated by the unruliness of it, how it seemed to have a mind of its own. He was an intriguing thing to behold, Laurence Price.

Loz was the world's most diligent listener, and Dean found himself drawn to his words of advice and encouragement, because they were always filled with such sincerity - Loz cared. Now, whatever he had to say, Dean wanted to hear it, even if it was only ever a small, passing comment. His silky voice carried itself hypnotically through the air and resounded endlessly within Dean's head; the sound of his comical laughter always managed to lift him out of even the sourest of moods. Loz was simply wonderful, from head to toe, inside and out, and Dean was definitely in love.

Just then, a text bleeped on his mobile from the bedside table at the opposite end of the bed. Dean groaned; he didn't want to get up to look. He knew who it would be from and tried to block out the details of the mess he had managed to get himself into. What was the devil doing, entangling the sleeping angel in his midst in his corrupt life?

CHAPTER 17.

The next morning, I woke up early…very early - about 5:00am - and it was still dark. Realising that what had just happened between us was not a dream after all, I just couldn't wait to open my eyes. Dreaming was such a waste of time when you could spend it lying there, watching the person you loved. No amount of dreaming could match real life, especially if what you normally dreamt about was snuggled up right beside you in the flesh.

Fully awake, and with the biggest grin smeared across my face, I turned to face Dean, who seemed to still be sound asleep, snoring gently - music to my ears. I watched him for a while, in awe of the masterful creation that was Dean Mackellar, and I studied his every detail above the covers, made lightly visible by the faded light of the moon; from his naked and well formed shoulders, which rose and fell with every breath, up his unusually slender neck. Then, I did something that, before last night, would have been inconceivably bold; I raised my hand and softly ran my fingers around his magnificent face, as if to trace him out. I felt so confident, so grateful that I could finally look at him with such intensity without having to flinch. Touching him was an added bonus.

The skin on his face was soft for the most part, bar the little stubble he had forming around his sideburns and the top of his lip, which felt curiously alien compared to the fair, downy hair I still had.

His nose was long and pointed - a good, strong nose. As was the same with his prominent forehead. The sheer chiselled-ness of him reminded me so much of one of those ancient Grecian statues.

Turning my attention to his eyebrows; they were fair and thin, but remarkably parallel on both sides of his face. I stroked them fondly with my thumb, marvelling at the light, bristly texture beneath my touch. I dared myself to explore further.

His heavy eyelids remained shut, as I then moved down to his mouth. His lips twitched as my fingers caressed them. Now, compared to the rest of his features, his mouth was not so remarkable. It was quite small, as were his lips. His teeth, too, in all honesty, were equally small and also a little crooked at the bottom. But those exact flaws were nice flaws; the kinds of flaws that, if anything, only ever endeared him to me more. Having flaws made him just that little more human, more attainable. Though no less perfect in my eyes.

I wanted to run my hands through the untidy mess that was his bed hair, which shone slightly from the natural grease in it and the messed up gel from the day before, combined with the reflection of the limited light on the mousey strands he had. I bit down on my bottom lip hard; it made him look so sexy and it was all I could do to control myself. He was a work of art, and a priceless one at that.

I continued staring at him for a long time, mulling over the night's events in my head, re-living every detail. Until suddenly, I was engulfed by panic and filled with doubt. What if he woke up and totally regretted everything? What if he blamed me for initiating the first move? Dean wouldn't have really wanted any of this to happen, surely? No, he couldn't have - he was far too *straight*. He would probably freak out and say that he had just got caught up in the moment, that what happened should never have happened.

I didn't think I could take that. I didn't think I could bear him saying those very words - it would only shatter my heart. I had to leave, to get out before he woke up, to prolong the inevitable. I wanted to hold onto the beautiful memory of our night together before it eventually became tainted by regret.

A few hours later at breakfast, everything was quiet. Bonnie had gone off early to the office and Dean hadn't yet come downstairs. Dad was in the kitchen making extra toast, and in the dining room it was just Nana and I.

I sat busily cutting up and buttering her toast, hiding my nervous shakes. I would have been sick all over the table if I wasn't trying to keep my mind concentrated on what I was doing. I gave Nana a weak smile as I passed her plate back to her, and she gave my arm a pat.

'Thank you, dear.' she squeaked in her underused voice.

"Welcome,' I mumbled, turning back, with a grimace, to my own food. I really didn't feel like eating.

'Are you alright, Laurence?' she ventured.

'Uh-huh, fine.'

Footsteps were heard, and then Dean appeared.

I looked up at him expectantly, and he gave me one of his signature cheeky boy winks in return. I beamed back, worries swiftly forgotten.

He said 'hello' to Nana, then reached for his seat. Out of the corner of my eye, however, I caught Nana watching me, and I quickly snapped myself out of my happy daze and continued eating with newfound hunger. Did she suspect anything?

As we headed noisily down the gravelled driveway on course for the school bus stop, I turned awkwardly to Dean. We hadn't spoken properly since last night, but, certain no-one was within earshot, I bit the bullet.

'Dean?'

'Yeah?' he answered earnestly.

'I love you.'

He stopped dead in his tracks and grabbed my arm to pull me back round to him. He just looked at me, and, for a split second, I didn't know what to expect. I almost regretted my brave admission as we stood gazing into each other, my heart doing laps, my feet fidgeting, as I waited for an answer. But he just carried on staring. Eventually, he opened his mouth to say something before stopping to look around. Then, as if fuelled by a bold and unyielding impulse from within, he took hold of the lapels of my blazer, pulled me a little way off the path - out of sight - and between the bushes.

He looked unwaveringly into my eyes again, stroked my jaw adoringly with his thumb and avidly kissed me.

'I love you, too,' he said breathlessly, resting his forehead on mine.

I felt like I was flying.

He sat next to me on the school bus that day and from then on.

CHAPTER 18.

'You know, I can't believe you're gay,' I thought out loud.

It was early that Sunday morning and I was lying with Dean in his bed - where I had been all night, as well as every other night for the past week.

'Why's that?' he said, rolling onto his side, the duvet falling away from his bare chest and revealing the subtle curve of his pecks.

'You just don't act it.'

He chuckled at that. 'How am I supposed to act?'

'I dunno…Camp, I guess.'

'You're not camp.'

'I'm no big butch guy like you, either,' I reminded him.

He sighed. 'Why do I have to be camp to be gay?'

'You don't. I guess it's just one of those preconception things,' I said absentmindedly, while pursuing my examination of the water mark stains on the ceiling.

'Yeah, well, just because I like guys, it doesn't mean I can't enjoy doing typical guy things,' he stated.

'Oh, I know.' I smiled at him in agreement. 'But talk about defying the stereotype, eh?'

We both laughed.

'I've always been curious to know, though,' I went on. 'How did you…well, *know?*'

'Know what?

I rolled my eyes. 'That you *liked* guys.'

He seemed almost hesitant to answer and wriggled uncomfortably where he lay. '…Ah, well, you know…had a thing for a guy…'

I wondered bitterly whether this meant he had had his heart broken before. 'Oh.'

'But then I met you,' he said quickly, caressing my face so lovingly that I felt the muscles relax. I must have looked tense.

I went back to gazing up at the ceiling, and jealously thought about this other crush of Dean's. No doubt he had been everything I wasn't - the epitome of masculinity. I decided it was probably best for my ego that I didn't ask for anymore details.

'What if I was more into sports and cars etc.?' I asked instead.

Dean frowned. 'But you're not.'

'I know I'm not, but doesn't it bother you that I don't really like to do a lot of the "typically guy things?"'

'You know that stuff's not *all* I'm interested in, either.'

'Yeah, but still...'

He laughed softly. 'Loz, I love you for who you are. You wouldn't be you if you were *that* conformist!'

I glanced confusedly at him and pouted. 'I don't know why you love me.'

With that, he became abruptly serious, as he lifted himself up onto his elbows and stared me down. 'Now, you listen to me, Laurence Price. You *are* a fascinating being. There's hardly a day that goes by when I don't think how lucky I am to even know you, let alone hold you!'

I could feel my face burning; the intensity of his words penetrated my heart. Though I guessed I would never fully understand why, it was clear from the sincerity of his tone in the things he said, and the, now, unmistakable gleam in his eyes whenever he looked at me, that I was as special to him as he was to me.

'I'll always want you,' he insisted, putting a cool hand back to my flushed cheeks. '*Always.*'

I stared back at him hard, drinking in his radiance and promises. My heart then spluttered excitedly, and I couldn't help but feel the need to pull him closer.

I kissed him full on the mouth, delighting in the tingling sensation that pulsated through me, and then whispered tenderly in his ear, 'Then I belong to you, Dean Mackellar. You and nobody else. Never forget that!'

'Never!' he breathed.

And that was that.

CHAPTER 19.

It was the beginning of December. Dean and I had been together secretly for a little over a month, and things were still in the honeymoon stage. I was so supremely happy that I couldn't possibly imagine feeling any other way ever again. Every waking moment was a blessing, particularly every moment I got to spend with *him*.

My senses now seemed powerfully heightened since the recent euphoric shift in my life. I was suddenly acutely aware of my surroundings, forever marvelling at things as day-to-day as the sun, the sky, the trees, the smell of fresh flowers etc...and as corny as it sounds, I was finally beginning to recognise their every poetic detail and significance - everything took on a whole new meaning. Life was a horribly cheesy fantasy, and I loved it!

Another reason for being in more of an elevated mood than I already was, was that Bonnie hadn't had much luck with house hunting - or so she said - and had been left with little choice but to book herself and Dean into the B&B for another couple of months.

Personally, I think it had more to do with the fact that she and Dad had been getting quite a lot closer lately. Seeing them snuggled up together on the sofa night after night watching telly was quite sweet, but of course, whenever someone interrupted them, they always pretended as if nothing was going on.

Dean didn't like to see it, though. He said it felt weird knowing that if things went too far with them, he and I could end up as *brothers*! But I never really believed it would get that far. I just couldn't sense the same kind of passion between them that Dean and I had, so I didn't let it worry me. In the meantime, I supposed Dad and

Bonnie deserved a bit of happiness together. I was just thrilled to know that I had Dean for a bit longer. It had really bothered me knowing that he and his mum were only temporary guests. Now things were working in everybody's favour.

It was currently early that Saturday morning. We were outside the village bus stop waiting on the 7:30am bus to take Dean into town. From there, he had a train to catch to Luton. He was going back to see a few old school friends – JayJay and Alyssa. And although he was only going for the night, even that absurdly short amount of time felt like a night too long to my captured heart.

I knew I would only mope around waiting on his return, so I made a conscious effort to book solid my weekend with plans with Zen and Frankie.

Although at school, to avoid suspicion, Dean and I hadn't had a lot of contact - with the exception of a million and one texts throughout the day (needless to say, mobile phone credit bills were through the roof!) - I had been kind of neglecting my friends outside of school recently. I knew it wasn't entirely fair or healthy to do that, so I was going to make up for it starting from today.

We stood in the freezing winter air, huddled beside each other for warmth. Though it's hardly easy to appear inconspicuous as a couple when: a) you're bitterly cold, b) your secret lover is standing so irresistibly close to you, and c) on top of that, they're also leaving you for an *entire* weekend!

'Do you *really* have to go?' I whined, still not wanting Dean to leave in spite of my own plans.

He sighed. 'You know I do.'

I huffed childishly, 'Oh, *fine*!...But you're only gone for the one night, right?'

He grinned. 'Yep, and then I'm right back here again.'

'Okay.' I smiled back, appeased. 'By the way, this doesn't mean I'm being overly possessive or anything. I just care, that's all.'

'Sure.' He laughed. 'And anyway, I have to be back tomorrow. We've got school come Monday.'

'Oh, yeah.' Of course we did. Love was making me stupid.

'So...Do you think I can sneak a quick goodbye kiss?' he muttered into his coat. His impressive eyes turned upwards at me, dazzling me.

'I would love that.' I beamed. If things were my way it wouldn't be quick, though. We still had four whole minutes to spare!

We moved inside the shelter. Fortunately, it was still quite dark out, and there was little to no activity on the streets. Nobody would even notice a pair of queers making out, discreetly tucked away in the corner of the wooden bus shelter.

I leant against the inside wall of the shelter and let Dean wrap himself around me. Anyone who did happen to look our way would barely see me behind him and his massive coat and tight arms. With an ever increasing need for constant gratification from Dean, I was becoming more and more daring in public these days.

'It's cold,' I chattered.

'Yeah, I kinda picked up on that, too.' He smirked and kissed me softly.

I hugged him closer to me and tried to push the thought of our impending separation out of my mind, while enjoying the electric pulses his lips sent through me as they reacted with mine. I never did get over the sensation.

After what barely felt like any time at all, he broke away from me.

'I wish you wouldn't kiss me like that! You're making me really regret leaving, now,' he chuckled between breaths.

'Hmm. Well, hurry back and you can have some more tomorrow.' I bit my lip seductively.

His eyes came alive with mischief. 'Oh? Maybe I *should* stay...'

I laughed. 'I'm the one who doesn't want *you* to go, remember? Besides, you'll disappoint your friends...and mine, for that matter!'

'Oh, *fine!*' he scoffed.

I laughed at him.

He glanced at his watch. The bus was now imminent, and so I begrudgingly let him lead me back out onto the roadside.

'You gonna be alright?' he asked.

'Of course. I'm spending the weekend with the guys - we're having a sleepover at Zen's.'

'Okay, cool. Just remember to be safe, Loz.'

I rolled my eyes. 'Oh, yes, because I hear sleepovers are fraught with all kinds of peril these days!'

'I mean in whatever else you get up to, Loz!' he said irritably, his expression wracked with real concern.

I thought then that I maybe had an idea as to what he was angling at, as my thoughts drifted briefly back to Jammy. Dean must have been hoping I wouldn't somehow bump into him while he was away.

Jammy hadn't been at school much since the incident back in October. My guess was that he had been vehemently warned by Dean to never come near me again if he valued either his life or a clean police record. He hated school, anyway, so it wasn't too much of a surprise to find him bunking classes. Though, conveniently, they tended to be ones I had with him, now.

I quickly erased the thought of Jammy from my head, like I had recently taught myself to do. I had come a long way in these past few weeks since, and I was now so content with life that it didn't do to dwell on darker times.

'I will,' I promised after a moment. 'You look after yourself, too, though.'

He pursed his lips. 'Naturally.'

Just then, the bus rounded the corner.

'Shit, it's here!' I grumbled.

He gathered his things and took a step closer to me, squeezing my arm affectionately as the bus squealed to a halt.

'Love you,' he whispered to me, facing away from the on-looking passengers.

A thrill always went up my spine whenever he uttered those words. I still couldn't believe how genuine they sounded.

I blushed - which even in the biting cold I'm sure is hard to do - and smiled toothily. 'I...you too.' - I was very aware of the weary-looking, but equally curious, passengers staring and waiting impatiently for someone to embark. But Dean seemed to understand, and winked knowingly.

It was fun, from time to time, being part of Suffolk's best kept secret - thrilling, almost. But sometimes, I couldn't help but think it would be nice to be as open and relaxed as every other couple out there. I wanted more than anything to throw myself on Dean right there and then, to really express my distress at his leaving.

However, I knew people around here were yet to catch onto the whole "alternative romance" scene. Country bumpkins always are a bit behind the times.

'Don't do anything I wouldn't,' I threw in for effect, as he hopped onboard. Though a sinister part of me hoped he got my hidden meaning behind that.

He sat at a window seat and gave a little wave as the bus started to drive off. My heart went with it.

I waved after him, vainly wishing upon hope that he would change his mind and dramatically jump from the bus, back into my waiting arms.

My instant loneliness was palpable. I felt suddenly very weak, as though only half of me was really there - the other half was on that bloody bus! It was a very helpless feeling, and I hoped it wouldn't be like this every time Dean had to go away. How would I cope?

I couldn't help but send the ridiculously cliché 'missing you already' text.

ℭ

Dean sat alone on the bus, listening to pointless gossip emanating from the mostly elderly passengers sat around him.

He wasn't going to visit JayJay Biggs and Alyssa Watson at all - they had near enough forgotten about him the minute he left Luton months ago. No, he was actually going to visit someone else. Someone called Alex Lowe.

He didn't like having to lie, but he hadn't known how else to handle the situation. Things with Loz weren't supposed to have got this far, but neither did he regret the choices he had made up to this point. It was just the inconvenience of it that he could do without.

Originally, Dean was only going to stay at the B&B for a little while - play along with his mum's new idea of happy families for the time being. He would bide his time, and then, finally, break free.

He would then go back to Luton, back to Alex, so that they could be together again. Then they would run away together, find jobs doing whatever they could, and live happily away from the prying eyes of nosy, narrow-minded neighbours and the backwards social circles their families moved in. Yes, that would teach the meddling pricks once and for all to ruin their happy existence, for separating them and for dragging Dean out here to the middle of God knows where in order to forget about the "silly, little whatever it is" he and Alex had had!

They had been good mates for years, he and Alex. Their mums had been best friends from way back, and so naturally the boys had grown up together. But one curious day, not too long ago, things between them took a different, more interesting, turn. They didn't think what they were doing was wrong, but they weren't naïve enough to think everyone they knew would be okay with it. However, in time, the two became careless in their affections for one another, and, sure enough, the alarm was raised.

The method of separation was a huge overreaction, especially in this day and age, and Dean felt wronged by how he and Alex had been subsequently treated. What they had had wasn't illegal - certainly not for the last half a century or more, anyway! He just wanted revenge of some sort, really. In truth, more than he actually wanted Alex; it was just the principle of it.

Then, on that fateful day he arrived at The Brambles, he met Loz. There was a spark. Something was there and he knew Loz had felt it too. Being with Alex had been great, but it was nothing compared. Alex had never really made his heart pound whenever he touched him, or even simply by being nearby. Dean was never more captivated than when he noticed things about Loz; the way his cheeks flushed whenever he got embarrassed - which was a lot; his hilarious laughter; the illusive dimple that appeared whenever he smiled; the way his puppy-dog eyes would widen and bore into you whenever he was worried about something…

Agreeably, he had been very fond of Alex, but Dean had foolishly mistaken this to mean love. It was, of course, not love at all, but purely lust. Love was what he knew now, what he felt for Loz. He had known that right from the very start, he supposed. The moment Loz had walked into his life, it was as if the missing piece of a jigsaw puzzle within him had been found; a missing piece he never knew was even missing to begin with.

He had to do it. He had to go to Alex and break it off, face to face – his old friend deserved that, at least. He would understand.

Just then, a text beeped from Loz:

Missing you already! X

Dean smiled warmly to himself. His tensed body instantly relaxed in one heaving sigh.

CHAPTER 20.

It was later that day, and I was at Frankie's.

I waited for her on her untidy bed in her über funky room as she rummaged through the accumulated mess on the floor around us for overnight things, throwing random bits and pieces into her heavily graffitied school bag.

'So, what's on the itinerary for the rest of today, then?' I asked her over Katie's noise next door.

'Nothing special. Bit of Christmas shopping in town, dinner somewhere, and then maybe we'll visit the vid-shop before we go back to Zen's.'

'Midnight feast included?'

'Definitely!'

It sounded good. Maybe not as good as a night in with Dean, but…no! No, stop it! I wouldn't even compare the two; it wouldn't be fair. Dean may have been my boyfriend, but Zen and Frankie were my best friends. They deserved just as much of my focus and attention as he did.

'How's Deano?' Frankie asked, attempting to rearrange the mess.

Frankie was the only other person who even knew about me and Dean. She had been sworn into secrecy, but to be honest, had she not managed to prise out a love confession from me, not even she would have known. Mine and Dean's relationship wouldn't exactly go down well in a school full of image-orientated, immature teens, and Dean was adamant that his mum shouldn't find out. He said it had something to do with her strong traditional values, and that it would just make life a hell of a lot easier if she remained in the dark.

'Yeah, he's good. I saw him off this morning,' I sighed, remembering.

'Aw, he'll be back before you know it.'

I nodded. 'Yep. But I'm all yours this weekend.'

'That's right. God, it's been too long!' I could tell she was insinuating at my recent absence from our group activities outside of school.

'I know, and I'm sorry. I'm a crap excuse for a friend,' I said guiltily.

No sooner had the words escaped from my mouth than she was already by my side.

'You're not a crap friend, hon. Just one who's very much in love - for the first time, too--'

'And *only* time,' I interjected.

'…Sure.'

I glared at her.

'Anyway, I know you've not ditched us on purpose. You're new at this, and you just need to learn how to manage your time better, that's all. Dean's as much a part of your life now as we are.'

I smiled up at her and leant my head on her shoulder. It was nice to have such an understanding person in my life.

'Besides,…we were here first,' she said, poking me teasingly in the ribs and getting up to continue packing.

I giggled. 'Damn right! Now, are we gonna get a move on, or what? Christ, we're only going for one night! I swear, it takes you longer than a *girl* to pack!'

She picked up a pair of dirty undies and threw them at me as payback. I swatted them away in revulsion.

'By the way, maybe you ought to think about explaining some of this *Dean* stuff to Zen, hon. He still doesn't know a thing,' she remarked.

'What? No! You know I can't.'

'Loz, he's your best friend, too. Maybe he'll understand. Especially with you having been so distant lately…'

'I'm making up for lost time now, aren't I? And anyway, not even *you* were supposed to know about me and Dean. You pulled it out of me, remember?'

'All I'm saying is, think about it,' she said, ignoring my protests and staring me down.

'*Fine*, I will,' I sulked, knowing I probably wouldn't win this argument. She did have a point, after all.

'You guys at least told your folks yet?'

'No!' I said before she had even finished.

'Why not? I'm guessing you two are serious now, right?'

I rolled my eyes in sarcasm. 'Yeah, but it's a bit more difficult with us, Frank.'

'It's the 21st century!' she insisted.

'Still, his mum's pretty old fashioned and we're living in the same house. Our parents don't need to think that we're probably sleeping together, as well,' I said hotly.

An impish grin crept onto her face. 'You've slept with him?'

'Off topic, Frankie!'

'Sorry.'

'The point is, regardless of the times, the idea of two young guys shacking up under one roof behind their parents' backs is not something we should probably broadcast.'

'I'm sure your Dad would be fine about it. The relationship bit.'

'My nana wouldn't be.'

'You don't know that,' she said.

'Frank, I've not just got to think about myself here--'

'I know, I know. It just sucks, that's all,' she huffed. 'I still can't believe you've managed to keep things a secret for all this time.'

I smiled playfully. 'Neither can I.'

We both laughed.

'So, you've slept with him, then?'

'Pack, woman!' I barked, throwing random items of clothing at her.

Zen lived about a mile away in Stuffham. Fortunately, Frankie's stepmum, Karen, was more than happy to give us a lift in her ancient something-or-other - a car that was so old, that all traces of its make had either worn away, or broken off.

Zen's family lived in a quaint little cottage with his zany mum and dad and little sister, Gem, at the very edge of the tiny village. Their bungalow home was more like a time capsule back to the

1960s, though. They had shag carpeting throughout; hideous, retro wallpaper; beaded curtains for doors; lava lamps and incense candles, which filled up every available table space; and there were beanbag cushions wherever you stepped. Even Zen's bed was a simple futon! The joys of having hippy parents, eh? It was like visiting the Brady Bunch, in some way - a family trapped in another time. Though, what was even funnier was that Zen's parents hadn't yet been born in the sixties!

Zen did his best to shrug all this off, but I knew he resented his parents for the way they lived. They didn't allow mobiles or computers for fear that that kind of "mindless technology" would "warp his fragile sense of expressive creativity;" they just about had a telly, but it was terrestrial only, and viewing times were limited to a strict minimum; and he had only recently managed to persuade them to let him have a DVD player - his only real luxury possession.

You could see the front door to the Stone residence a mile off; it was painted hot pink with daisies all over it. And in the front garden, there was a commemoration to Scooby Doo in the form of a rather psychedelic VW van. Frankie and I couldn't help but smile at the sight of it all. Poor Zen.

'Hi, Mrs Stone,' we said in unison as his mother, Coral, opened the door to us, sporting her long tie-dye robes. I thought I spied the painfully shy Gem clinging to the back of her mother's long garment.

'Hello, my dears,' she cooed, letting us in and giving us each a single daisy - popping Frankie's in her hair for her. Next, she group-hugged us; I never quite got over the shock of that whenever I visited. 'How are you? It's been far too long! I trust all is harmonious with you and your families?'

'Err, sure, yeah,' Frankie said, notably a little confused at Coral's choice of words.

'Zen, my sweet, your darling friends are here,' Coral turned and sang back into the house. Gem, still trying to remain hidden, seemed to move around her mother in shared motion with the sway of the robes.

Zen emerged from the distractingly busy-wallpapered living room, coming to rescue us from his eccentric mother. His baggy shirt was sprinkled with what I hoped was water.

'Thanks, Mum - hey, guys!' - he half-heartedly raised a hand at us in recognition at our arrival - 'Erm, by the way, Mum, the waterbed's sprung a leak.'

Coral sighed. 'Oh, dear, not again! I'll have to get your father to repair it when he comes back from his meditation class.'

I bit the inside of my cheek hard, choking back the laughter.

''Kay. Well, come on guys. Let's dump your stuff and get out of here,' Zen said impatiently, sensing our awkwardness and leading us towards the sanctity of his simple bedroom.

Once finally back outside to present day, we walked to the village bus stop and waited on the 1:10pm bus into town.

'Your mum's sweet, Zen.' I smiled.

'She's a bloody airy-fairy nightmare, that's what she is! Her and Dad!' I knew how easily embarrassed by them he was, and I suppose you couldn't blame him. 'Why couldn't we have done this sleepover thing at one of your houses?'

'Because I'm not allowed boys over to stay the night,' Frankie said.

'And it's your turn,' I added.

'Look, Zen. Everyone's embarrassed by their parents,' Frankie said gently, rubbing his arm in a comforting way.

'At least none of your families are a bloody blast from the past!' he spat.

'At least you have a real family!' I contended.

Okay, so judging by what I had just seen of Zen's home life, "surreal" was probably a more fitting word to use, but still, I was a right to a certain extent. At least he had a mum and a dad who were happy together...and alive! That was more than either Frankie or I could boast.

Frankie's real mum lived in Spain with her Latino lover, and so she only ever got to visit her once a year – usually in the summer. 'Any excuse for a holiday,' Frankie would say, but I knew, deep down, it upset her having such limited contact with her mum. And meanwhile, she lived in a dumpy estate in a village with a mostly bad reputation with her, apparently tone deaf, sister, her stepmum, and a dad she barely saw, anyway, because he worked nights as a security guard at the local sugar beet factory.

As for me, I knew very few people who could empathise with my lot in life, and it was now more than ever that I thanked my lucky stars that I had Dean. With that thought, my heart gave a twinge in longing.

'What we *mean*, Zen, is that things could be worse,' Frankie said more tactfully.

He quickly understood what we were hinting at, and abruptly stopped his moaning after that.

Our shopping spree in town wasn't exactly enthralling, but then Christmas shopping never really is. Being students, it didn't help that we really couldn't afford much, either.

I was getting tired of never having enough money for things, especially now that I wanted to get something special for Dean. He had a nice watch in mind, but the particular one he wanted was a very trendy, brown leather-strapped, digital watch, and it was by no means cheap!

Dean had recently taken up a part-time job as a weekend butcher's assistant at the Hobden village butchery - a place that prided itself in selling the finest local produce. He hated it, and constantly complained about how all he ever seemed to do was make restaurant burger orders and do the washing up. He hated the smell of the raw meat that lingered on his fingers long afterwards, as well. Still, at the end of the day, it was money and he needed it. He was doing well with his driving lessons and hoped to pass his test soon enough. Therefore, he also needed to start saving up for a car. If he had enough left over after that, he said, he would definitely buy the watch.

I was desperate to be able to get it for him, instead. But £70 was *a lot* for me, and I wasn't sure if it was too indulgent. I mean, we had only been going out for a little over a month. I marvelled at how fast the time seemed to have flown.

Unfortunately, I had only managed to save up £30. And even though I did get a £20 allowance every month from Dad for helping out around the B&B, money was just too easy to waste away. I also had to bear in mind that Dean wasn't the only person I had to buy for, and I wouldn't be due anymore allowance until January.

Note to self: get a weekend job soon!

We did a spot of shopping in Bury town centre's token alternative fashion style shop, Sundance, so that Frankie could buy herself a pair of killer-healed kinky boots - something she had been saving up for. Her sense of outrageous fashion taste never ceased to amaze me. She had decided that whatever money she had left over from today's shoe purchase she would spend on the rest of her family's presents… which, of course, didn't end up amounting to much. I wondered out loud why she didn't just ask for the boots for Christmas, but she insisted that, either way, she knew all she would get was another pair of bed-socks.

Zen had been instructed by his mum to buy his sister a particular doll for Christmas, to be given to her "from Santa." EcoEllie had been newly introduced to show young girls that there was an alternative to aspiring to a world of pink - green could be far cooler! Personally, I thought it was political correctness gone a tad overboard. As it was, Zen's sister could expect almost the whole range of EcoEllie merchandise come Christmas morning, ranging from her mini anti-global warming protest kit to her cutesy gardening equipment range, which included a complimentary bag of seeds for an assortment of vegetables.

As for me, other than buying Dad a fancy new potato peeler, I didn't get anything. I was still struggling for ideas for people, and I didn't really want to buy more until I knew exactly what to do about Dean's gift.

'There's still a good few weeks left 'til the 25th, you know. Plenty of time,' I reminded the guys as they peered disparagingly into my single shopping bag.

By about 5:30pm we were hungry enough for dinner, and so decided on The Vines pub - the place Dean and I had gone to only few months back, where we had met up with the super slags, Holly and Donna. I shuddered involuntarily as I remembered them. I hadn't been at all impressed to learn that Dean had merely used them in order to tease me at the time, either. Anyway, during the day, The Vines was also known to serve good, cheap family food before its rowdier regulars arrived for their evening binge drinking sessions.

We found an empty booth and shared-looked at the only menu on the table.

'Think I'll have the cottage pie,' Zen mused.

'The Vines chicken burger meal for me,' I announced.

'Ooh, garden salad!' Frankie squealed.

Both Zen and I raised an eyebrow at her.

'What? It's healthy! And in case you haven't noticed, I'm getting a little chunky these days. I need to shift a few pounds.'

'Oh, bullshit, Frank!' Zen exclaimed.

She shot him a glance, a flash of annoyance in her willow-green eyes.

'I mean, I like you the way...' he stopped himself, and then coughed self-consciously. I could see his cheeks redden as he heard himself speak. 'I mean, you look fine to me.'

Her eyes sunk back into their sockets. Her face now almost the same shade as Zen's. 'Yes, well...' she said quietly, 'maybe I will just have the burger meal, instead.'

I sat back, smirking. This was one of the many subtle but awkward moments the two of them shared in my presence.

'I'll call the waitress over, then, shall I?' I said coolly, sticking up my hand for attention.

A girl came over, who couldn't have been much older than us. She was quite pretty; cream-faced, lightly freckled and her curly, fire-red hair was pulled tightly back into a ponytail. I saw Zen's jaw drop ever so slightly, and felt Frankie twitch uncomfortably beside me.

'Hey! What can I get you guys?' the waitress sang cheerfully.

'Erm--' Zen gawped at her.

'Two Vines chicken burger meals and a cottage pie,' Frankie answered quickly for him, an edge of impatience in her tone.

'Sure...and drinks?'

'Cokes all round, right?' Frankie asked, though without really looking at us for confirmation.

I agreed anyway, but Zen didn't seem to hear her - he couldn't keep his eyes off of the waitress.

'Three cokes, then, please,' Frankie said shortly, staring vexingly at the stupid expression on his face.

'No problem.' The waitress smiled and left us to it. I smiled after her, half wishing I could leave with her, too, knowing only too well that I was sitting next to a ticking time-bomb. Frankie did not look happy.

The atmosphere was expectedly tense for a moment.

'She was nice,' Zen said crassly. He was oblivious to Frankie's irritation.

'She didn't say much,' she pointed out tartly, looking away.

'Didn't she?' he replied, brushing a strand of untamed hair away from his bespectacled hazel eyes.

Oh, God, Zen! Shut-up!

'No, she didn't!' she snapped.

He eyed Frankie warily, deliberating whether or not to chastise her for her tone.

I looked at both of them and decided that invasive third party action *was* necessary. This was supposed to be a fun-filled, happy weekend with friends. Arguments were not on my agenda.

'Lord, I'm starving!' I moaned theatrically. Though I mentally kicked myself for not having thought of something more diverting.

'She *was* pretty, I suppose,' Frankie carried on. 'If you like that sort of thing...'

Zen chuckled as he leafed through the dessert's section of the flimsy-looking menu. 'Wouldn't kick her out of bed.'

I wanted to kick *him*!

'Urgh!' Frankie protested.

'What?' He looked at her innocently, smiling to himself.

'You're a pig, you know that?!' she said shrilly, her voice having steadily risen a few octaves.

As expected, a few heads turned, which embarrassed me. 'Frankie, *please*!' I hissed. This had the potential to get really gritty

'*What*?' she retorted.

'*Keep your voice down!*'

'I *am*!' she practically shouted. '*He*'s just being a male chauvinist, that's all. I'm entitled to feel a little bothered by it.'

'What?! I'm not being chauvinistic!' Zen cried. 'So I think she's cute. Big deal!'

'You just go about it in a grossly blatant way,' she sniffed, sitting back and folding her arms.

'Oh, leave it out, Frankie!' he growled.

I stared pleadingly at them both. 'Guys, *chill*.'

Just then, I noticed our drinks were on their way. But it wasn't the pretty red-headed waitress who brought them over - thankfully! This time, it was the barman. He looked to be in his early thirties, balding slightly, though not wholly unattractive, I surmised. Frankie must have thought so, too, because she sat up straight and shone her most brilliant smile at the unsuspecting man. I saw a flicker of something in her eyes, and I could tell she wanted to try something out.

Her sudden shift in mood hadn't escaped Zen's notice, either, by the looks of things. Out of the corner of my eye, I could see him narrowing his eyes at her, trying to scrutinise her behaviour.

'Here you are, guys,' the barman announced happily, placing the drinks expertly on our coasters.

'Thank you,' Frankie answered in a velvety-soft voice, fluttering her eyelashes at him. She didn't take her eyes off of him, even after he had smiled back and walked away.

'Okay, what was *that*?!' Zen snorted, once the barman was out of earshot.

'What?' She tilted her head at him, feigning ignorance.

'You know what!'

She shook her head and replied obstructively, 'Nope, I really don't.'

Now *his* face was annoyed. 'You were flirting with him!' Zen accused.

I groaned. 'Please, guys, just give it a rest! You're gonna make me lose my appetite.'

'So what if I was?' Frankie spoke over me, clearly enjoying her slice of revenge. 'I thought he was kind of *cute*.'

Zen appeared a little put out by this, but he wasn't stupid; he knew Frankie was only trying to spite him.

'Loz is right, Frank; just leave it,' he said quietly, scowling and distracting himself by tearing at the corners of his drink's coaster.

Seeming satisfied that she had, at last, got her point across - whatever the point was - Frankie did then settle down, and the rest of the meal went off without too many hiccups.

Although there may not have been anymore confrontations,

neither was it easy to miss the two of them glaring at each other across the table from time to time, or occasionally see their eyes wandering after the restaurant staff, as if to deliberately provoke the other one.

Truth be told, Zen and Frankie were known to bicker a lot. But then, never quite as heatedly as today. At least now the obvious was screaming them both in the face, I supposed. Things would come to a head soon.

I rolled onto my back and stared up at the blackened ceiling.

It was late Sunday night and I was home in bed. My weekend with Zen and Frankie had been okay, but the outburst over yesterday's dinner had left things between them a little raw. Afterwards, for the most part, it felt as though I was the one doing all the talking, trying to encourage things back to normal. We ended up renting out a pretty terrible slap-stick American comedy and going to bed early on the horribly uncomfortable waterbed. There had been no midnight feast, and Frankie had insisted we leave Zen's early this morning.

'Oh, well,' I thought. 'They'll be back to their old ways tomorrow, I'm sure of it.' They just needed a day or so to get over their awkwardness around each other.

The rest of today had been spent getting any outstanding coursework done, but even when Dean wasn't here, it was hard to concentrate on anything else but him. At least he would be home soon, and I couldn't wait! I had tried my hardest not to think about him this long weekend, to dedicate my time and thoughts fully to my friends, but I couldn't deny the anticipation I felt for his impending return. Every hour that passed brought him closer to me.

With it being Sunday, his trains were ludicrously delayed, so my guess was as good as his as to when he would arrive home. Of course, the already useless Suffolk bus service gave up after 4:00pm, so his mum was on call to collect him whenever he got back into the station in town.

Bonnie had been on edge all week; I wondered why. She really didn't want Dean making the journey down to Luton. I guessed it was because she was simply worried about the lengthy and confusing trip he would have to endure. Suffolk was, after all, in the middle of nowhere, and public transport to and from here was notoriously crap. In spite of Luton being almost literally next door to us, he would have to travel right out to Cambridge, down to London and then back on himself up to Luton; all of which added unnecessary time onto an already strenuous journey.

He kept me updated frequently on his whereabouts by text message, but after 11:00pm, Dad had forced me to go to bed. But I just lay there waiting, wide awake and waiting for my Dean to come back to me.

Amidst thinking about how wonderful Dean was, I must have eventually drifted off. Because, the next thing I knew, my bedroom door was quietly opened and a dark figure came plodding in and squeezed in bed beside me. I snapped myself out of my sleepiness, as I recognised the delicious scent and felt the familiar shape of the body pressed up against mine. I pulled Dean closer to me, wrapping myself tightly around him, and inhaled. My heart danced.

'You're back,' I said quietly, eyes still shut and enjoying the moment. 'What time is it?'

'It's 1:00am,' he whispered. 'I didn't mean to wake you. You missed me?'

'Does a bear shit in the woods?'

He laughed quietly. 'I suppose so.'

'Then you suppose correctly.' I tilted my head upwards, waiting for him to accept my 'welcome home' kiss. He did, lowering his lips and relinquishing them to mine; a powerfully magnetic force welded us together.

I ran my hand over the contours of his lightly toned chest through his shirt. He then pulled away from my lips and let the tip of his nose follow the soft curve of my jaw before planting gentle kisses down the length of my neck.

'I take it…you missed me,…too?' I breathed erratically.

As he slowly slid down me, I could feel the tremor of his eager breath on my skin, while his masterful hands worked over me teasingly. Every sensation he unleashed within me practically consumed me, as I surrendered my body and soul to him once more.

He lifted his head up briefly through bouts of heavily aroused breathing. 'Does a bear shit in the woods?'

I giggled, pulling him back to me. I gently parted my lips and greeted his again, slowly at first, with each preceding kiss becoming ever fervent.

If the old saying was true, that being in love meant that I was a fool, then so be it.

CHAPTER 21.

Dean was a monster - a disgraceful excuse for a human being. Or so that's how he felt.

Every time he looked in the mirror, now, all he could see was an incredibly stupid, sleazy lowlife. He wanted to hit himself, to punish himself in anyway possible. It enraged him to even look his own reflection in the eyes. 'You inconceivable bastard! You don't deserve what you have!' he thought aggressively of himself. He had betrayed Loz. He had done the worst thing anyone could ever possibly do to the one person they loved more than life itself. What's more was that he didn't even know how it had happened in the first place. Everything had been such a blur. One thing was for sure, though; that was the last time he would ever see or speak to Alex Lowe again - the cruel, selfish, psychotic freak that he was!

It had been a week since he had got back from his trip to Luton, and Dean was getting tired of acting as if everything was okay when he was around Loz. He had to admit, though, he was doing a good job of it. But his whole body ached with the guilt. He so desperately wanted to say something. He knew he had to, but for some reason, there was always something in those warm, gentle eyes of Loz's that made him think twice about it. He didn't like the idea of hurting him, and if he ever found out…well, Dean couldn't even bring himself to think how Loz would react. Things made sense now that they had found each other, and Dean was terrified of the inevitable pain and suffering it would cause them both if ever the truth came out. He knew it was unbelievably selfish and morally wrong not to say anything, but he didn't want to lose Loz. The very idea of it made his stomach turn.

Today was predictably cold, and Dean was going into town to buy Loz's Christmas present. It was going to be the best damn Christmas present Loz had ever had! He thought about maybe buying a symbolic ring - hell, he had enough cash saved up from his Saturday job to afford something like that! Maybe a ring was a little excessive after only having been out with Loz for such a short space of time, but Dean was more than convinced that they were meant for each other. This ring would be a token of his irrevocable love and devotion. In spite of the irony of its symbolism, it didn't make it any less true; Dean knew he would never even dream of hurting Loz like that again, whether consciously or not. It would symbolise a new start for him, at least, even if Loz was none the wiser.

Just then, a text flashed from Alex. A lump, the size of a golf ball, formed at the back of Dean's throat. He had deleted him from his contacts' list, but he still recognised the number. Hesitantly, he read:

I'm in town. We need to talk. It's important. A x

'What?!' Dean thought out loud.

He considered honouring the promise he had made to himself, to never speak to Alex again...but curiosity plagued him. What could Alex possibly want now? He had already done his best to ruin Dean's life!

Dean stared at his phone a while. He *had* to know what Alex wanted...then he would definitely vow to never talk to him again.

Dean scrolled for the number, pressed it and it rang. He felt some of the leftover anger resurfacing. There wasn't a lot left to say that hadn't already been said, and yet, as he waited for Alex to answer, he couldn't help but feel himself getting angrier still. He felt like he had to say something more, as if whatever he had said before hadn't done his loathing and disgust any justice. But he knew he would only end up repeating himself, and so thought it best to keep the conversation short and sweet, no matter what Alex had to say.

'Dean?' Alex answered anxiously after the fourth ring.

'Where *exactly* are you?' Dean asked curtly, his temper already dangerously high.

'I'm in Bury town centre...I got the train this morning.'

'Go home, Alex!' he demanded.

'No. Look, I've come to talk to you--'

'There's nothing left to say,' he growled.

'There is, there's something I...something I didn't--'

Dean looked quickly about the street to check that there was no-one in sight before he uttered his next sentence. 'Enough, Alex – we're over! I love Loz. I've told you that a million times!....And anyway, after what you did to me,...how you've caused me to betray him! You're dead to me, you understand?!' he fumed, his fists clenching and turning white.

'Dean, please, you've got to listen to--'

'I don't want to hear another word from you, Alex...ever! You've done enough fucking damage! Just do me and favour and PISS-OFF!' With that, Dean cut him off. Hopefully for good.

He shook with rage where he sat in the shelter. A thick cloud of condensation swirled around him as his breathing became faster and louder. Loz's present would just have to wait until next week, he thought, as he headed tensely back towards the B&B.

❧

Unbeknownst to Dean, he had had an eavesdropper throughout the whole of his phone conversation with Alex.

Jo Reiner had been on her way to call on Cyndi - the lovely, beautiful Cyndi Langham. She and Jo used to be friends...sort of. They didn't exactly hang around in the same crowds, but they had known each other all their lives, living in the same village and all. And to top it off, Jo was, rather inconveniently, secretly in love with her – she supposed she had always been. Ever since Dean had arrived on the scene, however, Cyndi only seemed to ever have time for *him*.

Cyndi was a hopeless case, Jo knew. There was absolutely no way Cyndi would ever be interested in her the same way she was in Dean. Because Jo was a girl and Cyndi was straight, and it broke her heart a little more each time Cyndi mentioned the *oh so gorgeous* Dean Mackellar in her presence. Cyndi was besotted with him, so Jo Reiner had decided she hated him!

But today, after thinking she had all but lost Cyndi to this apparent knight in shining armour, Jo now had the juiciest piece of gossip she had ever heard.

Dean and Loz. How unexpected. How precious!

A wicked smile snaked across her thin lips as she stepped out from the holly bush near the bus stop, where she had hidden out of sight on hearing Dean's suspicious exchange. Maybe things would work out well for her, after all.

CHAPTER 22.

The next day, after school, as everyone got off the bus, Jo took the chance to corner Dean. Cyndi was *hers*, and things needed to happen soon if she was ever going to get over her silly infatuation with him.

As was routine, the ever popular Dean would exchange a few quick goodbyes with the rest of the Hobden school kids before running off to catch up with Loz. But today, Cyndi was keeping him there a little longer than usual.

Jo began walking her own way home, but once she was sure no-one would notice her anymore, she dived behind a nearby tree. She then strained her ears to listen in on Dean and Cyndi's conversation, peeking round the side of the wide trunk.

'So, erm, I just wanted a word, really,' she overhead Cyndi say tentatively, obviously thinking she and Dean were finally completely alone together.

'And what's that?' his husky voice was calm, if a tad distant.

'Well, you see…Dean, we've known each other a little while now, a-and…well, I think we've become quite close…' Cyndi babbled, 'and so I was wondering, you know, if…possibly…you and I, you see…we…'

Dean frowned and crossed his arms impatiently. 'Cynd,' he stopped her, 'what's up?'

'I…well…' she started again, then sighed, apparently giving up. 'Oh, come on, Dean. Don't make me say it. You must know where I'm going with this.'

Jo knew exactly what was on the tip of Cyndi's tongue, even if Dean didn't, and it was absolute agony to know it.

'I really don't, Cynd,' he replied ignorantly. He was either really bad at social cues, Jo thought, or he was doing his best to play on Cyndi's shyness in order to evade her looming question.

'I like you, Dean,' she blurted.

He didn't look surprised. 'I like you too, Cynd.'

'No,' she huffed, exasperated. 'No, Dean. I *like* you.'

Jo winced. That smart.

Dean's face showed no emotion. This obviously wasn't news to him, either. But then again, to any outsider, it was fairly obvious that Cyndi Langham had the hots for Dean Mackellar. She didn't hide it well.

'Cynd...' he started ruefully.

'And I was wondering if you'd maybe like to go out sometime,' she persisted anyway, sensing a losing battle.

There was a brief pause. And for a second, Jo was scared that her audibly bounding heart would give her hiding place away.

'Cyndi, I *do* like you...But...'

She looked crestfallen. 'But...' she repeated.

'*But* not like that.' He smiled weakly at her as if that might make her feel better. 'I'm sorry, hon.'

'No, no, it's okay,' she flapped, her voice going squeaky. Jo recognised the tell-tale signs of oncoming waterworks. 'It's really fine, honest.'

'Look, this doesn't change a thing between us,' he assured her.

'Oh, no, of course not!' She nodded fiercely, putting on a brave face. 'Right. Well, I suppose I ought to get going home...I'll see you tomorrow, yeah?' She patted him on the shoulder and walked away quickly, no doubt intending to get as far away as possible before the tears began to fall.

In spite of Dean being the cause, Jo struggled to refrain from chasing after Cyndi at that moment, to comfort her in her time of need. 'But at least she can now begin to understand the pain,' Jo reasoned with herself - unrequited love was an old friend of hers.

Dean gave a massive heave where he stood before moving off in his own direction...which was also the direction of Jo!

This was it, she told herself.

She wouldn't move from her spot just yet, though. Instead, she tried to relax her posture where she waited awkwardly up against the old, weather-beaten tree, to ready herself.

'Hi, Dean,' she called out as he passed her unsuspectingly.

He jolted on the spot and rushed a hand to his chest, swinging round to see her standing only a few feet away. 'Christ, Jo! You scared the shit out of me!' he half-chuckled, while gasping for air.

'Yeah,…sorry about that,' she said unrepentantly. She gave him and his heart a moment. 'Just a quick word, if you don't mind.'

He moved towards her, visibly a little confused at the request. The two of them had never spoken together alone before. 'Sure,' he breathed. 'What is it?'

As she had feared, Jo became momentarily stumped for words. 'Oh,…well, it's nothing, really…' She looked past him, deep in thought. Now how should she phrase this next bit? She had been working on it in her head all day; she should know by now. '…Just this one thing.'

'Yes?' Dean blinked, waiting.

'Mmhm…well, it's you, you see,' she remarked casually, feeling the words finally coming to her.

'Me?' His eyes boggled. 'What have *I* done?'

Her face grew deathly serious. 'You *exist*, Dean. That's what you've *done*.'

The look of puzzlement on his face deepened. 'What?' he muttered.

'You've ruined everything!'

'H-how, exactly?'

'Cyndi's in love with you,' she stated, though she cringed at her own words; they were still hard for her to digest.

He looked at her as if she might be crazy.

'You came and she fell in love with you.'

He snorted at her, finally encouraged to fight back 'And how is that *your* problem?'

She took a deep breath before she opened her mouth again. She knew then that Dean would be the first person, other than herself, to know how she really felt about Cyndi. 'Whatever affects Cyndi, affects me.'

'How?'

146

'She's mine, Dean!'

'Eh?'

'I had Cyndi all to myself before you arrived. Things were going great...'

He continued staring blankly at her before eventually breaking out into disbelieving laughter. He had, at last, cottoned on to what she meant. 'Oh…Oh, I get it!'

'Stop laughing!' she snarled.

'You *like* her, don't you?' He smirked.

'Just shut-up!'

'Okay, okay.' He recomposed his face and, with some effort, became serious again. 'Just one thing, though. If things between you two were so "great," how come I never see you hang around together?'

'We *used* to!' she stressed. 'But then, like I said, you sauntered in and spoilt it all!'

'For God's sake, I'm not even interested in Cyndi like that, Jo!'

'Yeah, I know you're not. You're far too interested in fucking Laurence Price!' she fired.

That silenced Dean once and for all. He looked as white as a sheet as he stared back at her in complete shock.

❧

'Ah, so that got your attention, did it?'

Dean didn't know what to say. He thought they had been careful, he and Loz. How did Jo know about them?

'You don't know what you're saying, you conniving cow!' He scowled. He couldn't bring himself to deny the accusation, though.

'Ah, but it *is* true, is it?' she simpered. 'And what about this *Alex*?'

A chill went up Dean's spine. Oh, Lord! What *had* she heard?

'Interesting fellow, from what I gather.'

He glared at her. 'What do you want, Jo?'

'Cyndi.'

'Have her!'

'And for you to be gone.'

'Wha--?'

'You heard…' She stared at him. 'Don't you see? It's not enough for you to just say you're not interested in Cyndi. She *loves* you, and unless you're gone for good - all ties cut - she'll never get over you.'

'But, but *leave?*' he spluttered.

'Yup.'

He thought for a moment. He could sense an ultimatum on its way. 'Or else…?'

'Or else I let slip about this little thing you and Loz have got going on.' Her smile was chilling. 'Either that, or the Alex thing. Whichever is more damaging, I guess.'

He could have killed her. But then he chastised himself for being so careless about his feelings in public in the first place. What could he do? He couldn't simply up sticks and leave, that would be crazy! Besides, Loz meant too much to him.

In the end, he decided to call her bluff.

'I'm not leaving, Jo,' he said with finality.

She looked a little peeved at that, but didn't argue further, obviously still believing she had the upper hand. 'Fine. Have it your way.'

She then slunk off towards home.

'Oh, but, erm, Jo?'

'Hmm?'

'If ever you do say anything…I might just find it necessary to let slip about this little thing you've got going on for Cyndi.' He smiled slyly, giving her a devilish wink. Two could play at this game!

Jo's eyes instantly grew wide with angst. He could tell she hadn't expected this. Maybe she wasn't as bright as she seemed.

'Won't Cyndi be surprised!' he sneered over his shoulder at her as he walked away.

೭౨

Jo weighed up her options in her head as she marched up the winding path towards the cottage where she lived. If she *outed* Dean, he would, in turn, *out* her.

'Shit!' she whispered, putting a hand to her clammy forehead.

This was not how she had planned things at all! Still, at the end of the day, she supposed she had to expose herself to some extent in order to get what she wanted from Dean.

Also, compared to his, her reputation was nothing. It wasn't like *she* had much to lose. Whereas, from the look of things, Dean would have a lot of explaining to do. That, at least, brought a smile back to her face.

She supposed she could always deny her feelings for Cyndi, too, if ever Cyndi questioned them. Jo loved her, but she didn't want things to be weird between them. Though unrequited affections were by no means fun, she reasoned that being able to remain quietly in love with her, while still keeping close to her, was about as far as Jo was likely to get. So long as she had Cyndi to herself in someway, she could make do without any extra perks.

She would, therefore, stick to the original plan.

'Prepare for a very messy *outing*, Dean Mackellar!' she chuckled maniacally to herself, picking up her stride.

'Hey, Cynd! Fancy doing something this evening?' Jo asked the object of her affections as they shuffled their way down the bus after school the next day.

Cyndi smiled at her. She had always thought Jo was a sweet girl, a very attentive friend, but they weren't exactly close - not anymore, anyway. Her almost complete disregard for personal boundaries was a tad off-putting, to say the least. 'No, thanks, hon. I've asked Dean to help me out with my Geometry notes tonight. Maybe another time, yeah?'

This infuriated Jo. Though, deep down, she supposed she knew Dean wouldn't have taken heed of her threat, given his own. 'Sure. No problem,' she replied with a false smile.

Oh, yes! Now was as good a time as any other. Cyndi wouldn't have plans with Dean for much longer if she had anything to say about it!

☙

'Look, I'll be back a little later. I said I'd give Cyndi a hand with her homework,' Dean said.

'But I thought you were taking me to Flame tonight,' I whined quietly, only too aware of the other students walking past me. Flame was Suffolk's only gay bar, and they were having a Christmas-style under-eighteens' night tonight. Dean and I were thrilled to finally have the chance to be out in public together...if only for the one night.

'I'll be back way before then. I'll try and only be an hour, tops,' he promised.

'Alright,' I grumbled. 'But couldn't she have asked for help from a teacher, or something?'

His expression was sympathetic; he understood how annoying I found it whenever Cyndi stole opportunities to flirt with him.

'She knows you're not interested in her, right?' I whispered earnestly.

'Yes.'

'Then why is she still bothering?'

He raised an eyebrow and he smiled crookedly. 'Can you blame her?'

I punched him playfully on the arm.

Just then, Cyndi leapt from the bus, followed closely by a serious-looking Jo Reiner. They were the last to get off. The other kids had disappeared off home.

'You ready, Dean?' Cyndi called to him.

Looking away from her, Dean rolled his eyes and I stifled a snigger. 'Yup,' he said loudly.

'Seeya, then.' I half-smiled, fighting the urge to kiss him, to publicly stake my claim over him.

Before I turned to move away, however, I noticed that, from the sheer severity of the expression on Jo's face, she really did not look happy. A storm appeared to be brewing within her, and she directed a viciously intended scowl at Dean. This annoyed me, and I felt instinctively protective of my, seemingly oblivious, boyfriend. How dare she look at him like that!

What I overheard next, though, pricked my ears.

'Oh, I thought you already had plans with Loz tonight, Dean?' she said loftily to him.

How did *Jo* know about *our* plans?

'Erm, no. Whatever made you think that?' He answered her. Though he sounded as if he was speaking through his teeth.

'Really? You see, I could have sworn…Oh, no, I'm sorry. It was *Alex* you had plans with, wasn't it?' she said.

Alex?

'What? Alex who?' Cyndi asked, not knowing who to look to in her confusion.

'I don't know.' Dean shrugged violently. 'I don't know what you're talking about, Jo.' This time, I definitely detected a hint of hysteria in his tone. What was going on?

'Oh, didn't you know?' Jo continued.

'Know what?'

'That he had plans with this *Alex*…Ah, no. Sorry, again. You're quite right, Dean, you don't have plans with Alex tonight--'

'*Jo!*' Dean hissed.

'--because you had plans with Alex a few weeks ago, didn't you? That weekend you were away in Luton. Surely you remember that, Loz?' She looked over to me with intimidating eyes.

I shuddered. Something was telling me I wasn't going to like what was coming next.

'*Jo!*' Dean hissed again more loudly.

'Yeah…didn't he tell you he'd been off to see his old--'

'*JO!*'

'--*boy*friend, Alex?'

Boyfriend?!

Mine and Cyndi's faces must have been mirror images of each other's.

Jo, however, looked very pleased with herself. 'Oh, yes, Cyndi. Didn't you know Deany, here, is a bum-boy?' she said calmly. 'From what I hear, his poor old boyfriend's been dying to know what he's been up to lately…' she smirked, again looking purposely at me.

Jo definitely knew more than she let on. My heart had practically deflated in my chest, and I could feel my face go green with sickness. Why on Earth was she saying all of this, anyway?

'What?! Shut-up, Jo!' Cyndi squealed in disbelief and laughed shrilly. But she only had to look at Dean's panic-ridden face to know there was some truth in it. 'Dean? What is this? Is what Jo says true?'

It was my question exactly!

'Oh, God,' he heaved. He was fidgeting and I could see beads of sweat forming above his brow. He dipped his head nervously, then looked up at both Cyndi and I, and gawped at us before eventually regaining some form of composure. He then turned on Jo with fierce eyes. 'Fuck you, Jo Reiner! Fuck you straight to hell, you smarmy shit-stirrer!'

I couldn't say or do anything. Lord knows I wanted to, but I knew I would only be putting myself at the epicentre of all this shit if I did. So, I just stood there, shell-shocked, and trying to take it all in, while also trying to swallow back the surge of bile that crept up my throat. Who was this *boyfriend*? Dean had mentioned a crush, but never a boyfriend. So much for me thinking I was special! Maybe all I was, was another notch on his bed post; and maybe wherever he went he found another sexually confused boy to torment with his irresistibly typical, gay-boy-wet-dream / jock-like ways before eventually sleeping with him. The anger and the hurt quickly began to rise up through me, steadily overtaking the urge to vomit.

'Dean, what the hell is going on?!' Cyndi demanded.

'Nothing, that's what, Cynd!' he snapped back at her.

'Then, what's this about a boyfriend?...Are you...gay, Dean?'

He sighed. 'Why does it matter to you either way?'

'Because...!' She stared at him.

He read the signal and shot back, 'We're not going out, Cyndi. I've told you already, I'm not interested!'

'So, you *are* gay, then?'

I could see the tears glistening in her eyes.

'Well,...not that it would probably have made a difference either way, but yeah, 'fraid so.'

With that, she turned on her heels and ran up the street in the direction of the park. I could hear her muffled sobbing in the distance.

'Cyndi...' Dean called feebly after her.

I continued to watch on, mentally orchestrating what I might say to Dean when I got my turn.

'Thanks again, Jo! I really must congratulate you on well and truly fucking everything up, you callus bitch!' Dean spat, giving her a hard shove.

But she didn't even bat an eyelid. She took it all in her stride and didn't retaliate. Instead, she replied with an evil grin stretching from ear to ear, 'You did that all on your own, Deany-boy. The way things were going, it was bound to all come out in the end – no pun intended.' She winked. 'I just helped things along a bit, that's all.'

She turned and strode off in the same direction as Cyndi, no doubt to find and console her.

'You're a fucking piece of shit, you are, Jo Reiner! You fucking muff-diver! Go on, go after your *sweetheart*!' Dean yelled, throwing a rotten apple from off the ground at her, only for it to narrowly miss her. She just cackled dismissively and walked on, anyway.

As soon as she was out of earshot, Dean quickly turned to me and pleaded, 'Loz, listen. It's not what you think--'

'I'm going to go home now, Dean,' I said rather coolly, finding my voice at last. I had decided I was not, unlike Jo, going to start something out in public for the whole of the village to hear. We were lucky in that we seemed to have been left conveniently alone, the four of us, throughout the outburst. But as absurd as it may sound, I could just picture the whole story thus far plastered across the front page of the weekly village gazette with an unflattering photo of us all quarrelling, courtesy of some undercover local geriatric journalist. 'I don't think I want to go out tonight anymore, to be honest.'

He started to walk after me. 'Loz, please listen--'

'*No!* You *don't* need to follow me!' I growled.

So, I carried on ahead, shaking with bottled-up rage.

Thankfully, Dean did not follow me. I knew whatever else he had to say wouldn't have made me feel any better. His reaction to Jo's outburst had said it all. I guess I shouldn't have been all that surprised, really. Somewhere deep down I knew all this had been far too good to be true. Like an unimaginably perfect dream turned nightmare, but a nightmare that had gripped a hold of my heart and was attempting to rip it from me.

Fortunately, no-one else was in when I got home - they had all gone out to see a play at the local theatre and would not be back until late, or so the note on the breakfast table read. I just ran straight upstairs to my room.

I was determined, for some reason, to keep from crying; it was the one thing I wanted to do the most, but knew I couldn't. I would not waste tears on this. I had had a very dramatic change in attitude in the short space of time since the revelation, and my silently festering rage encouraged a previously unknown strength in character from within, thus overruling any other emotion. Dean was a bastard, and the fact that his true colours had come out now was a good thing.

At any rate, I had coursework - lots and lots of it, and it really did need a good seeing to. I had been constantly putting it off in favour of spending more time with Dean. However, I could now think of no better time than to really sink my teeth into it.

Later that night, after having spent a gruelling session at my desk and done, I thought, a rather thorough job, I heard a light tap on the door. I knew who it was and I took my time getting up to open it.

Dean was leant against the door frame, picking at the paintwork. He gave me one brief guilty look before turning to his hand at work. I just stood with my arms folded. Looking at his sheepish stance, his beautiful face, made me thaw a little, though. I didn't want to be angry, but he had wilfully deceived and humiliated me.

'Loz.'

'Yeah?' I harrumphed.

'I'm really, really, *really* sorry.'

'Yeah?' Was that it?

'Can I *please* come in?'

I didn't answer. Instead, I slowly moved away and went to sit on my bed. Dean came in and closed the door. A few silent moments passed, giving me more time to truly reflect on why it was I was so ticked off.

'Why didn't you say anything?' I started impatiently, tired of the suspense.

He answered almost in a whisper, 'I didn't know how.'

'So you didn't think that telling me about your other current boyfriend was maybe something you should have run by me before you started fucking me, too?!' I spat. It didn't half feel good to finally get that out!

'Loz, I--'

'I can't believe you! You know, it was like a dream come true when I realised you were as interested in me as I was in you. But I guess I should have known better than to believe I was the only one you had on the go, right?'

'Loz, I'm not like that, I swear! But this *thing*.' He gestured between me and him. '*Us, we, it* wasn't *supposed* to happen.'

I winced. That hurt a lot. 'But it did happen.'

'Yes, it did, and you know what? I wouldn't change any of it!' He looked seriously at me, but I refused to believe him.

'You still didn't tell me about *him*, Dean! He's the only reason you went back to Luton the other week, isn't he? You weren't with your "mates," JayJay and Alyssa. You were with *him* the whole time. This, this…whatever his name is.'

'Alex,' he said meekly, lowering his head in shame.

There was a pause.

'And did you sleep with him?'

Again, silence.

'Dean…Did you, or did you not, sleep with Alex?'

'…Yes.'

It was like someone had slapped me across the face and stabbed me in the chest with a rusty knife. Dormant tears bubbled fiercely up to the surface and I turned away so that he couldn't see me weakened by his admission.

I stared unblinkingly at the far wall. I inhaled deeply, trying hard to hold back the tears in my eyes, which threatened to spill out of their sockets. '…I thought you'd always want me…'

'I do!'

'No, you can't want me as much as you say you do when you went with someone else at the same time!'

'Loz, that's not--'

'Just get out.'

'Please, let me explain!'

'Explain what? How you're a lying, cock-hungry player who can't keep it in his pants long enough between fucks?!'

'That's not--'

'No! No explanation is necessary. FUCK YOU, DEAN! Fuck off back to Alex! Go on!'

He stood for a while, clearly stung, but obviously wanting desperately to say more. Eventually, thinking better of it, he turned and left, shutting the door gently behind him.

Right on cue, the tears I had been denying began to stream unrelentingly down my face.

I sat numbly for a few moments before realising I was actually going to be sick. My insides retched and I couldn't breathe. I ran to the sink and heaved furiously between bouts of heavy, inconsolable sobs.

Fucking Dean Mackellar! I wish I had never fucking met him!

CHAPTER 23.

It was about 2:00am and I was in bed, tossing and turning in frustration, unable to get the devastating image of Dean and his *precious* Alex together out of my head. I thought about Alex. I thought of how much better looking he probably was, and much more deserving of Dean's time than I evidently was. It killed me, and my pillow was now thoroughly drenched in salt water.

There then came a scuffling noise from across the landing, and the rustle of something being slid under my door. A letter. The light footsteps outside faded away as Dean - I could only assume - went back to his room.

I stared at the letter from where I lay for a long time. I wanted to know what it said, but at the same time, I already knew the worst of it and I just couldn't bear the details right now. He couldn't possibly justify his cheating on me, no matter what. Anything else he had to say would only be a load of grovelling.

I got out of bed, and instead of trying to read it, I picked it up and contemplated ripping it up and throwing it away. But I decided that no matter how much he had hurt me, I simply couldn't. I may not have wanted to read the letter right then and there, but at the same time, I knew I would one day regret not knowing what it said if I did throw it away. I was caught in a bind.

Eventually, I decided to house it in the top left- hand drawer of my desk for whenever I felt I would be strong enough to stomach his excuses.

I then went back to bed and silently cried myself to sleep.

I didn't come out of my room for a long time. I pleaded ill to Dad

- who didn't need much convincing, seeing how pale and drawn I looked - and I flatly refused to see anyone, even ignoring my phone. I may as well have been ill, as I felt like death, anyway.

I felt all empty and achy. My head span with past conversations, of good times Dean and I had had, which all the while only made things worse. The only thing I can find to describe what it was I was suffering from is, quite literally, a broken heart. Dad called it a fever and left it at that, and persisted in doting on me with food trays and medicines; all of which I gladly took in the vain hope that they might dull my emotions as well as reduce my pains.

I spent the days lying awake in disbelief of everything that had happened. I hated Dean for what he had done, but at the same time, I couldn't stop loving him for who he was. In the end, however, the perfect little dream world I had created of the two of us together was gone in that blink of betrayal, and I was confident I would never be able to forgive him for that. I was a love fool who had been royally fooled!

After some in depth thinking, I came to the inevitably difficult conclusion that I wasn't the first person to have had their heart broken and I would by no means be the last. And so, after spending the best part of a week in mourning, I finally felt strong enough to venture out of my cave. I still continued to keep my thoughts to myself, though, and I consistently refused to look at or even voluntarily talk to Dean, as I knew it would only send me over the edge again - I even went as far as to delete his number off of my phone! He needed not to exist to me, now, and henceforth I only ever acknowledged him in front of company. Even then, though, I kept the conversation light and my eyes averted. But when Dean was forever trying to corner me to apologise for the umpteenth time, that did make life living with him all the more unbearable. Fortunately, after a while, and much to his obvious dismay, he began to take the hint and leave me well alone.

Once back at school again for the last few days of term before the Christmas break, I noticed Cyndi moping around a fair bit. As far as I was aware, she hadn't blabbed about Dean's secret. I guessed she thought it too humiliating to admit to the world that she had fallen for a cleverly disguised, promiscuous homo. I felt exactly the same.

I even made it clear to Zen (not that he knew much, anyway) and Frankie - with my dagger-like glowers whenever he came up in conversation - that Dean was now a no-go area for me.

It helped that I knew where he would be at each time of the day, too - both at home and at school - and, like I used to do with Jammy, I lived life around him.

CHAPTER 24.

Christmas was a non-event for Dean and I, and it was the first Christmas I had had where I didn't feel remotely festive. I just wanted to stay in bed until after New Years.

Obviously, I hadn't got Dean a thing in the end, and after I sent back the pleading Christmas card he had posted under my door in pieces, I guessed Dean had thought better than to buy me something, as well.

Bonnie and Dad danced around all day, merry as anything. They hadn't declared themselves officially, but it was pretty obvious to the outside world that they were an item, now.

Dad had mischievously placed the mistletoe in the most inconvenient place - the dining room doorway - which gave him and Bonnie ample opportunities to kiss each other without it being considered too weird, just because it was Christmas. However, it wasn't something Dad normally put up each year, so I didn't expect it that morning when I begrudgingly came down for Christmas Day brunch.

It was an unlucky coincidence that Dean happened to be just leaving the room as I entered. Of course, everyone whooped and howled at the very idea of the two of us having to kiss each other. My cheeks burned fiercely with the embarrassment of the situation. We stood minutely in indecision. I hadn't been this close to him in a few weeks, and his proximity unleashed a powerfully confused wave of emotions over me. I couldn't look directly at him for fear that I would either head butt him or kiss him more passionately than was strictly appropriate for a mistletoe kiss. The thought of his intense eyes on me was enough to soften some of my resolve, though. I knew he wouldn't need to be asked twice to kiss me back, even if it was in front of everyone else, and I had to admit, I was sorely tempted.

'Oh, it's alright. Of course you two don't need to do it,' Bonnie giggled piercingly, as if purposely interrupting something. I snapped back to reality. 'It was just a silly game between John and I, after all.'

Dean mumbled a quick 'Merry Christmas' to me before fumbling past.

As I edged into the room, I became suddenly light-headed and quickly made to grab a chair to sit on before I swooned. Luckily, nobody was paying much attention to me to notice, allowing my face time to regain a healthier complexion.

The rest of the day was nothing special. Dinner was so-so, seeing as my appetite for food had diminished considerably of late, and my presents weren't all that spectacular, either - materialism was the last thing on my mind these days.

I had to act my way throughout the remainder of the holidays like that, carefully ignoring Dean whenever and wherever possible. Just because twas the season, it didn't mean I would forgive him.

CHAPTER 25.

The end of February. I had lived torturously side by side my ex, Dean, for almost three months, now, and things were still tough. Valentines Day had been the toughest by far. The day had never meant much to me up until then. In fact, like many cynical singletons, I just saw the whole thing as an excuse for hallmark companies to boost their sales. But this year, now that the word *love* had taken on a new meaning in my life, St Valentine really was rubbing it in my face!

Thankfully, I didn't see Dean for any of it. He had gone off somewhere on his own, probably to corner some other poor, gullible and repressed lad, I thought resentfully. Though I knew he was most likely just wallowing in the fact that I wouldn't permit him near me on the most romantic day of the year. All the same, I allowed myself a few tears that day.

With the New Year school term, also came ever more work preparations for the final GCSE exams in May. This particular weekend, near the end of February, I was concentrating on some primary research for my Art project on The Swan.

Ms Lethersby, my Art teacher, had suggested I 'really go out and look at live swans, to get a better idea as to their shape, size, texture and movement,' or whatever. Frankly, I would rather have had a lie-in. I wasn't altogether keen on wasting my Saturday in the middle of a freezing park staring at swans. But hey, it had to be done… apparently. So, after raiding through the bread bin and stuffing all my Art equipment into my school bag, I trekked over to the small village park.

For a Saturday, it was strangely deserted, bar a few dog walkers. Though I guessed that with it being so cold, people were sensibly opting to stay tucked up indoors today. I was, in someway, glad of this; I had been feeling pretty self-conscious about the idea of standing around gawping at the swans all week. I was a teenager feeding the birds, effectively – talk about embarrassing! With winter in full swing, I didn't even have the excuse of full, leafy trees or bushes to inconspicuously hide behind, either.

Luckily for me today, the river running through the village park was a) not frozen, and b) entirely littered with birds, including swans. Spring was in the offing for them, clearly. I cheered silently, realising I might get back home sooner than I had thought. The fact that there were so many birds did, however, make it more difficult to isolate the swans. I threw bread in aimlessly in the hope that I might catch their attention. But only the geese and mallards came. They were fast getting on my nerves, too, and were ever persistent, following me down the bank as I chased after the one swan closest to me. Soon, I ran out of bread and I hadn't even managed to get a close-up snap shot of a single one!

Bitterly disappointed, I stood around for a little bit hoping that swans could secretly read minds and would humour me a little by swimming over at least a couple of metres towards me. But the laws of nature were against me on that one.

'Bastard things!' I hissed loudly. I had only been there twenty minutes, but it was already turning out to be harder than I had originally anticipated.

I sat down on a grassy patch by the bank, feeling deflated. I didn't have the patience for this; it seemed wholly unnecessary. I needed more bread, but I couldn't be bothered to go back home to get it - not if I couldn't stay there. In the end, I got out my big sketchbook and started doing random doodles from what I could see of the swans from a distance. It was quite infuriating, as I really needed the close-up details. I thought again about turning back and maybe trying again tomorrow, but knowing my luck, the swans wouldn't still be here. Sunday was a day of rest after all, and it probably stretched to mean birds as well - even they couldn't possibly have the energy to flaunt their feathers gracefully *everyday* of the week.

There was a sudden disturbance in the water patterns, and I could hear light paddling. This was weird, because as far as I was aware, there was no boating dock nearby. This was only a very narrow river.

The paddling grew noisier as it came closer, and I could see it was already starting to upset some of the birds. This was not good for me, but all I could do was wait it out.

The small rowing boat eventually came slowly into view, and I was surprised to find that I thought I recognised who was rowing. Then my stomach plummeted; I realised I knew exactly who was rowing it.

'Loz?' I heard the instantly recognisable voice calling out breathlessly to me.

It was Dean. He knew I would be here.

Art or no, I wasn't sticking around. It had been far from easy, ignoring Dean all this time, but I had managed it. Of course, it still hurt like hell, but I just pretended he didn't have a face anymore, which actually helped quite a bit…in spite of his angel's voice. I had to get on with things, I had told myself. I had to make it through the days. I had better things to do than to soak every handkerchief, tissue and pillow around with my heartbroken tears.

Even still, I knew I would, somehow, have to acknowledge Dean again one day soon, especially if he and Bonnie were going to be living with us indefinitely. But not now. Now was still *too* soon.

I got up to leave. In hearing my frantic rustling as I packed up my stuff, Dean looked over his shoulder. Seeing his head move round, though, I quickly turned mine away from him.

'Loz, don't be like that. *Please.*'

What he was doing, I could tell, had some ridiculously romantic gesture hidden behind it, and, had things been on better terms, I would have no doubt lapped it up. The truth is, I wanted to be able to love that he was doing this, because a large part of me did. But that part was growing dangerously strong every second I lingered there on the river bank. He was very clever, I would give him that.

I started to move away. I had to be sensible. I would be stronger, much, *much* stronger.

'Loz!' he called out in exasperation.

'You deciding to come and surprise me on the river in a dinghy doesn't change anything, Dean,' I shouted back coldly behind me, eyes firmly shut so as not to accidentally look at him.

'Loz!…Okay, but wait, you dropped--'

But I tuned out the rest, putting in my earphones, and headed for home.

Sod the swans!

My head ached for the rest of the day. Thoughts and desires battled against logic. I did everything possible to block Dean out, like I usually did whenever he particularly got under my skin; I did my homework with loud music blaring out of my speakers, while the telly played on in the background. I also decided to skip dinner, again – I would grab a snack later on when Dean wasn't at the table.

At about 7:00pm, a knock came at the door. I froze in my seat, turning down the music.

'Who is it?' I asked tentatively.

'It's Dad,' came a voice.

I breathed a sigh of relief. 'Come in.'

He smiled as he walked in. 'Hey, you.' He closed the door behind him as he entered and went and sat on the end corner of my bed. Something pulled at my heartstrings as I thought back to when Dean would sit exactly there.

'What's up, Dad?'

'You weren't at dinner again today,' he said, concerned.

'Yeah,...sorry. I did tell Nana, though. I'll probably go make something in a bit.'

He sighed. 'Loz, what's wrong?'

'Nothing,' I lied as convincingly as I could. Typically, though, he read me like an opened book.

'There is, Loz, don't lie. You've been getting skinny, you know. You're not starving yourself, are you?' he rambled on parentally.

I almost guffawed at that. He didn't know how way off he was.

'No, Dad, I'm not starving myself. I'm just not hungry...Besides, I've got a lot of work to do.' I motioned at the stack of text books in front of me.

'You're exams are ages away!'

'Dad, it's practically March and my first exam is in May! I've got *a lot* to do before then...'

He shook his head. 'Okay, fine. I suppose I should be glad you're taking you're exams seriously. But you've definitely not been yourself lately, and I'm worried about you--'

'Well, don't be.'

'--And another thing,' he carried on, anyway, 'are you and Dean not friends anymore?'

He was crossing dangerous territory here.

I tried to do my best to act nonchalant, even though my chest was fluttering wildly. 'We're okay,' I lied again.

'It's just that the two of you used to be so close. Now you hardly ever seem to talk. Has something happened between you?'

Just then, I noticed Dad had something in his hand, and I found a window of opportunity to change the subject.

'What's that you've got there?' I said brightly, pointing at the concealed object.

He frowned, visibly annoyed by my evasiveness, but answered me, anyway. 'Oh, this? Yes, Dean wanted me to give you this back. He saw you in the park earlier and said you dropped it. He said he tried to get it back to you, but that you were too far ahead and couldn't hear him. You be careful with things like this in future; cameras don't come cheap!'

He placed the little, electric blue-coloured, digital camera beside me on the table.

There was a pause.

'It's definitely Dean, isn't it,' he stated. 'Loz, whatever's the matter, you can tell me. You know that.' He held my gaze.

He was beginning to get on my nerves. 'It's nothing, Dad!' I said hotly.

'I'm just saying...' He held up his hands in defeat, sensing my irritableness. 'I'm just saying, I'm here.'

'I know!'

He got up then, finally taking his cue to leave.

'*Whatever* you want to talk about--' he reemphasised, eyebrows raised.

'--Then I know who to come to,' I finished for him.

As the door shut behind him, I leaned back in my seat and exhaled deeply. Parents!

Then, remembering the camera, I reached for it and looked it over. I swore at myself for almost having lost it, and then groaned at the prospect of having to repeat my excursion tomorrow.

I switched it on to make sure it still worked after its ordeal, and, as I did, a beautiful close-up of a swan appeared on the little coloured screen. This puzzled me, as I knew full well that none of the pictures I had taken were *this* good.

I flicked through to find even more of the same or similar images. Swan after swan in clear-cut detail, and from every angle and possible position.

As it dawned on me, my eyes began to well up. Dean had done the work for me.

I quickly switched the camera off and pushed it away from me. I then tried to control my breathing as I gulped back the tears.

I sat in contemplation for a moment, taking in what I had just seen. This was an even more ridiculously romantic gesture than his row boat stunt, and I was filled, again, with such conflicting emotions; I wanted to run to him; I wanted to hit him; I wanted to shout at him; I wanted to kiss him...

But, as I calmed down, I established with myself that I was, indeed, more angry than anything. I thought, how dare the pillock do something so wonderfully kind as this when he knew I was trying to get over him!

So I rushed out the door and stormed across the landing to his room. I had my fist ready to strike the door, when I forced myself to stop and rethink my actions before I did or said something I might soon regret. While it was true that Dean had done something really lovely today, it wouldn't be enough to redeem him. I decided I would simply say thank you for the help, as was only polite, but nothing more.

I held my breath as I knocked, my heart pounding so hard against my ribcage that it hurt.

'Yeah?' Dean's voice came.

I opened my mouth to say something, but only air came out.

'Hello?' he called again, this time more anxiously. I could hear him moving around.

Before he had the chance to open the door on me, however, I turned on my heels and hurried back to my room.

I thought I would be strong enough, but clearly I wasn't.

CHAPTER 26.

Dean opened the door in time to see the back of Loz disappear behind his bedroom door. Though crestfallen, he knew better than to chase after him. So, he, too, retreated back inside his room.

He stood with his head against the back of the door and, almost at once, lost all feeling in his legs, sliding to the floor. He trembled violently as silent tears streaked down his cheeks. He had never felt so stuck, so beaten.

He had done everything he could possibly think of to win Loz back, but nothing had worked. It was clear, now, that Dean was beyond redemption in Loz's eyes.

There was nothing left to it, he thought. He had to leave. Lord knows he didn't want to, but it wasn't doing either of them any good, him still living here. Loz wanted to move on, and Dean would just have to respect that, no matter how much it pained him.

The only problem was, he and his mum were booked into the B&B until the end of May - his mum's budding relationship with John Price had meant they were staying on longer than they had originally anticipated. Although, both she and Dean had furtively hoped that their stay at The Brambles would eventually turn into a more permanent arrangement.

But enough was enough, Dean decided. He had made his bed and now he would just have to lie in it. He knew exactly what he had to do now, too; something very simple that would have him and his mum gone by morning, if necessary.

Later that night, once he had collected together his thoughts, he tiptoed across the landing to his mother's door. He hated how there was always a door in the way of everything in this house, but then he appreciated the fact that this kind of conversation required a level of privacy. Loz mustn't know; the less said, the better - a goodbye would no doubt be more than was bearable. Besides, Dean knew his mum wouldn't exactly take too kindly to what he was about to tell her.

'Mum?' he called, rapping softly.

There was a squeak of bedsprings and the sound of rustling sheets from within. Then came his mother's out-of-breath, and slightly agitated, voice. 'Y-yes, Dean? What is it?'

'Can I come in?'

'*No!*' she shouted, and Dean almost jumped away from the door. 'I mean,...can you give me a few minutes, dear? We--I'm just in the middle of something--'

We?

'This is kind of important, Mum. I need to speak to you, now!'

'*What does he want?*' came a muffled male voice that Dean recognised at once.

'Mr Price?'

What was John doing in--?...*Ew!* Actually, he didn't want to know.

There came a loud shush. 'L-look, Dean, darling. Let's talk more in the morning, shall we?'

This really couldn't wait. Dean didn't have the mental strength to wait until morning. He had to say it all now while it was fresh in his mind, and before he had time reconsider. And he figured John would have to find out at some point, anyway, so...

'I have to speak to you, *now!*' Dean declared as he waltzed in, determined. He wisely averted his eyes.

'Dean!' his mother squealed, mortified, and gathered up the covers around her. She tried her best to hide most of John with a pillow.

Dean rooted himself to the floor and crossed his arms stubbornly.

'Dean! What is this?! Get out!' Bonnie hissed.

'No! I have something to say, and I'm not leaving until I've said it. You're not gonna like it, I'm afraid...'

The look on her face didn't change, although her tone, at least, did. 'Alright, you're scaring me, now. What's the matter?'

He glanced at John, who was trying to discreetly slide even further under the covers. Dean couldn't think of a worse situation to say what he was about to say, but he held his nerve. 'You may as well hear this, too, Mr Price. It concerns Loz…'

❧

As I braced myself for breakfast the next morning, I was struck by how quiet the house seemed. I came downstairs to find both Dad and Nana sitting at opposite ends of the breakfast table in silence.

Nana was looking at Dad with a worried expression, as she shakily spooned porridge into her mouth. I went to look at Dad more closely. He was slumped over his own bowl, running his spoon around the rim absentmindedly. He also had huge, purple bags under his eyes. I knew the look all too well. Had he been crying?

'Dad? What's wrong?' I asked frantically, pulling up a chair next to him.

He simply smiled a false smile back at me. 'Oh, nothing, mate. Just tired, that's all. I didn't get much sleep last night…'

Then another thing struck me.

'Where are Mrs Mackellar and Dean?' I asked. It was late in the morning; they should have been up by now.

Dad got up and started putting the surplus crockery away in the side dresser. 'They've left, Loz.'

Left?

'Wh-what? What do you mean *left?*'

'In that they're not here anymore.' He shrugged languidly.

It was as if I had had the wind knocked right out of me. I knew I hadn't necessarily liked having Dean around all the time since he had broken my heart, but I was still shocked to hear the news all the same. It was just so sudden. If I had at least been forewarned, I would have had more time to psyche myself up to the idea.

'Oh,' was all I could muster. But this was a good thing, I tried to tell myself unconvincingly.

'Yeah.'

'Wh-when did they leave?' I stammered on.

'Very early this morning.'

Dad looked back at me empathetically. In that very instance, that look of intuition, I could tell that, somehow, he knew about me and Dean. If nothing else, the poorly masked, agonised expression on my face must have been a dead give away.

'Oh,…okay,' I breathed, still flustered. 'And, erm, where have they gone to, exactly?'

'Not sure. Somewhere far, though,' he said, robotically clearing away more breakfast things. He eventually disappeared into the kitchen.

I sat at the table for a little while, chewing on my lower lip as I processed this new information. This was definitely a good thing, I kept reminding myself.

'Laurence, dear?' Nana squeaked at me anxiously, snapping me out of my reverie. 'Are you alright?'

She stretched a frail hand across the table in a subtle attempt to comfort me.

'Hmm? Oh, yeah,…Yeah, I'm fine.' I nodded vigorously, getting up at last. '…Erm, I don't feel much like having breakfast at the moment. I think I might go for a little walk…Try and work up an appetite, you know.'

I left before she could say anything else.

The sky was clear, and I headed back towards the park. I needed some space to breathe. Everywhere felt claustrophobic.

'This is definitely, completely and utterly for the best, Loz.' I mumbled out loud to myself, as I power-walked down the lane.

I knew I was just being silly. Dean and I were no longer together, and hadn't been for a while now. His leaving made perfect sense. No more temptation, and I could finally move on. It was all good.

But it didn't feel good. I was, of course, still hopelessly in love with him.

Once I reached the park, I found a soft, out-of-the-way patch and collapsed into a heap on the ground. The grass beneath me was still a little damp from the previous night's rain, and not even the oddly warm and penetrating, late-morning sun was able to ease the incredible tension that overwhelmed me. I still felt terribly uncomfortable, still felt as though I was suffocating on my own heart.

It was the finality of it all that I was finding hard to take. I had no choice now but to finally let him go. There would be no goodbyes.

I burst into tears at the realisation that I would never see Dean's magnificent face, or hear his deep and tender voice ever again. The pain of knowing that everything I had once cherished was all gone, was excruciating.

I felt as though a large part of me had disappeared right along with him.

CHAPTER 27.

Contrary to how I had felt at the time, my wounds did slowly begin to heal as time went by. And, as expected, new tenants arrived and, if only temporarily, helped fill up the gaping hole the Mackellars had left in all our lives.

I can't deny there weren't moments of weakness, when all I could think of was *him*, and how our lives would be if we were still together etc. But I guessed the love I felt for Dean would take a considerable amount of time to get over. I couldn't push it, but I could do everything in my power to help move it along.

My exam revision, in particular, proved a very welcome distraction. I would get up early, go to school, be with my friends, work my arse off, come home, and then work my arse off some more until I literally fell asleep with my head in a study guide. If I was lucky, I would maybe have time to squeeze in a meal or two, as well. It was far from healthy, I know, but at first, when I picked up on this effective outlet, I relished the idea of no longer having time to think about Dean. Finally, there weren't enough hours in the day left to be alone with my thoughts.

Up until that point, I had grown to resent the idea of going to bed. Going to sleep was fine, it was the *bed* bit I didn't like. After a busy day of diversions, there wasn't a lot to do in bed except try to sleep, and that left room for thoughts and images of the very person I had been burnt by to fill my mind. Then would come the processing of old conversations, visuals of passionate moments together, the wondering as to whether or not I had made the right decision to leave him....

Studying until I dropped ensured that none of this happened.

It was an exhausting way to live, but it was the only method that seemed efficient enough in coaxing my heart back to some form of normality. And despite the constant tiredness, I was once again beginning to feel more positive about the direction my life was going in. Hopefully I would pass my GCSEs, I would move up to sixth form college, and from there I would eventually move on to university and study to become a famous artist!...Or something to that effect. Either way, I refused to let this *Dean* business drag me down. He would not be the be all, end all of my existence.

All was going relatively well until one day, on a typically chaotic study evening in mid-spring, surrounded by towering piles of revision guides, mock papers and note-makings, I was rummaging around for my protractor in my top left-hand desk drawer when I came across Dean's unopened letter.

My gut clenched painfully at this small reminder of him.

I remembered hiding it away for a time when I felt more ready to listen to his rambling excuses. And amidst all the emotional drama, I had almost completely forgotten about it. But here it was again, after so many months, in front of me, still unopened, secrets still intact. Curiosity finally got the better of me. With Dean and his mum gone, maybe it was the knowing that this was the only connection I had left with him - though tenuous as it was - that was drawing me to it. Besides, in spite of my initial reaction to rediscovering the letter, I was sure I had moved on enough to bear whatever he had to say.

I moved away from the desk, perched myself on the edge of my bed and impatiently ripped open the envelope. A tightly folded wad of lined paper fell into my lap. I picked it up, unfolded it and eagerly read.

Loz

Look, I know you're pissed off with me, and I would be too if I was in your shoes, but you've got to hear me out! Alex <u>was</u> my boyfriend. He and I were together before my mum dragged me all the way up here to Suffolk.
He was the real reason why we moved. He was also the reason why my dad left - couldn't tolerate the fact

that his only son was into guys! Mum, on the other hand, wouldn't give up on me. She still holds onto the hope that one day I'll turn round to her and say I was pretending all along.

Anyway, I was going to leave here as soon as I could - escape back to Luton, back to my life with Alex. We'd planned to run away together, get jobs somewhere and live happily ever after etc. But then I met you. The very day I met you, you changed my perception of the world as I knew it. The more I got to know you, the more I realised that what I'd had with Alex was, in comparison, nothing. I'm in love with you, Loz. You know that. I've never felt like this before, and you're the only one I ever want to feel this way about.

When I was sure you felt the same way about me, I made a point of going back to Luton to see Alex, to tell him, in person, that it was over between me and him.

Alex had no idea of my intentions prior to my visit, and so he was, naturally, keen to continue things from where we left off. But I explained to him that that was no longer the reason why I was there. I suggested we went out for a drink somewhere to chat, where I quickly told him about you and how much I cared for you. He was obviously upset by it and thought I was bluffing at first, but he knew I wouldn't lie about something like that. It became pretty clear, even to him in the end, that I was deadest on you and only you.

The rounds kept coming, and, soon enough, I was drunk. The next thing I knew, it was morning and I was in Alex's bed. I assumed the worst had happened when he stirred next to me and started laughing. I just know he planned it all; he took advantage of me, Loz, while I was intoxicated, and he didn't even try to deny it.

I feel sick to the core knowing that I've betrayed you. And I know drunkenness isn't exactly the most winning excuse for what's happened, but honest to God, I can't

remember a single thing from the rest of that night, Loz!
Please believe me when I say that whatever did happen, it
wasn't the real me. I could never intentionally hurt you.
Needless to say, Alex is out of my life for good, now, and
I only hope that you can, somehow, find it in your heart to
forgive me.
Know that I love you and always will.

Yours <u>forever</u>

Dean

A familiar numbing sensation began to creep over me. I didn't
know what to do with myself. Did I believe any of it or not? A part
of me wanted to. Did it make a difference either way? That same
part wanted it to. With Dean gone, though, and me with no way of
contacting him anymore, I wouldn't even be able to confront him
about it. He no longer even went to my school.

I stopped myself there, however, before I got too carried away
with my thoughts; I had been doing so well, recently. And anyway,
even if what Dean had written *was* the truth, it was still a lot of
baggage to take onboard. I didn't have the time or patience at this
crucial stage in my life to worry about relationship drama. No. I
would stand by my decision. I would be a far better, far stronger
person for it in the long run, I was sure.

At least I knew a little bit more about myself, now, I concluded;
I could be thankful to Dean for that if nothing else, for bringing me
out of my shell. At least I *had* loved, and it had been everything they
had said was, if not more. But now, I was just going to have to chalk
it up to life experience.

My heart had lost the battle over my logic, and slowly, but
determinedly, I placed the letter in my waste paper basket.

'Enough, now,' I told myself.

CHAPTER 28.

May: Eek!

Exams were to begin at the end of the month, which was only a couple of weeks away. Though my first exam was French oral and I was sure I would ace it, my compulsory curricular modules I was less sure of. If I wasn't allowing myself to miss Dean, I could at least miss his occasional tutoring. I really didn't know how I would get through it all, to be honest.

'Not long now,' Zen heaved as he stretched out his long limbs on the playing field one break time. The day really was too nice to be stuck indoors stressing over mock exam papers.

'Oh, God! Don't, Zen!' I covered my eyes and fretted. 'I'm so not ready.'

'Ah, you'll be fine,' Frankie said distractedly, picking at the daisies and beginning to make a chain. 'I can't wait for the prom, myself.'

Frankie was one of those irritating students who never seemed to do any work and yet still managed to come out top of the class. If her attitude in lessons wasn't so deplorable, she would have no doubt been a crowned teacher's pet by now.

Normally, I might ask her to help me with my revision, but her method of tutoring lead a lot to be desired for. She got too easily frustrated with me whenever I didn't understand something the first time round; it was all so obvious to her, whereas trigonometry and the science of the electromagnetic spectrum were things I needed to be slowly talked through. I was a conscientious student, but studying did not come easily for me.

'Oh, shit, yeah, the prom!' Zen half-laughed. 'I keep forgetting about that.'

To be honest, if it weren't for the constant poster reminders around the school, I would have forgotten all about it, too. Understandably, exams seemed to be the only thing on anybody's mind these days… except for Frankie, of course.

I frowned. 'I can't believe the prom is more important to you than your final exams, Frank!'

'It's not *more* important. I'm just looking forward to it, that's all. I need a break from all this studying business' - (Like she even studied!) - 'And besides, I have the perfect dress lined up. I can't wait!' She beamed.

I sighed and asked, 'So, you got yourself a date, then?' I knew she hadn't. That was normally something she would have made publicly known by now if she had.

Predictably, and sulkily, she answered that no she hadn't.

'But that doesn't matter. I can still go with you guys.' She reached over and took my hand in hers. I managed a smile back. She knew I wouldn't be at all looking forward to prom. It would be an unnecessarily painful reminder that Dean wouldn't be there to chaperone me.

'Err, yeah…about that,' Zen then piped up.

'Yes?' Frankie eyed him warily.

'I've kinda already been asked by someone.'

Her jaw dropped comically and she spluttered, '*What?*' before coughing self-consciously and relaxing her forehead. 'I mean,… what?'

'Yeah,…erm, it's Julie Riggs,' he mumbled, his cheeks now flushed.

Frankie looked as if she might die from revulsion. I was just as shocked as she was, actually.

'*Julie?*' I stressed.

Zen's face showed no sign of returning to its normal shade. 'I know, I know. It's just that…well, she asked.'

'So, if she asked you to jump off a bridge, would you do it?' Frankie spat.

I rolled my eyes. He had woken the beast!

He grimaced. 'What? No! Don't be stupid, Frank! You know that's not what I meant.'

I could see her knuckles whiten as she clenched her fists; the damaged daisy chain gradually fell apart as it poked out either side of her balled hands.

'Okay, Zen, but it *is* Julie we're talking about,' I reemphasised.

He shrugged. 'I think she's alright.'

'That arse-kissing, little goody-two-shoes?! She's positively the most boring, most plain person on the face of the planet!' Frankie fumed.

Zen then sat bolt upright. He didn't look like he had any patience for her tantrums today. 'Hey! Just what *is* your problem, exactly?'

'I don't have a problem!' she retorted.

'*No*, she doesn't have a problem, Zen.' I glared at Frankie in warning. 'You're right, though. There's nothing wrong with your going to the prom with Julie if that's what you want.'

'Thanks, Loz,' he said to me appreciatively.

'Well, I still say it's wrong! We were all going to go to prom together. You knew that!' Frankie argued.

'Oh, but it would have been okay if you'd had a date?!'

'Nothing's been set in stone, Frankie,' I reminded her.

'Shut-up, Loz!' she snapped.

I was stung by her ferocity. 'Oi!'

'You know what your problem is, Frank?' Zen's temper was flaring. ''Cause I do! I know you *like* me, and I know it bothers you that I see other girls.'

She was stunned into silence. I was, too.

He then hastily got to his feet and dusted himself down. 'I'm sick and tired of your jealousy!' he continued. 'For God's sake, Frank! Don't punish me just because you're too afraid to tell me how you feel!'

With that, he stormed off back towards the main school building.

'Zen...' I called out after him. I was torn as to who I should go to comfort first. But as I turned to look at Frankie, I saw that she was now doing a fairly good impression of a statue, her face locked in a state of shock.

I touched her hand gently, as if to instil some life into her. 'Frank?...Hon, are you okay?'

She slowly turned to see me, eyes shimmering with a thick layer of tears. 'Oh, dear God, Loz,' she mouthed.

I threw my arms around her as she crumbled into me.

'I'm so sorry I snapped, I…' she choked.

'Shush, shush,' I muttered as I rubbed her back. 'It's okay.'

'No,' She shook her head, her already untidy, auburn hair ruffling against my shirt. 'No, it's not, Loz. It's really very *not* okay!' she wailed.

'Hmm….Well, I suppose you could say that at least everything's out in the open, now,' I soothed. '…And about time, too, if you ask me.'

Her head shot up, and her eyes narrowed in question. 'Wha-? Wait a minute…you, you *knew*?'

I bit the inside of my cheek to suppress a smile. 'Erm, yeah… 'fraid so.'

'Oh, no!' she hiccoughed.

I laughed. 'Oh, come on, Frank, it's really not that bad.'

She stared at me incredulously. 'How can you say that? You saw how I was, how he reacted!'

'And my guess is he *likes* you, too.'

'Ha! If that was true, he wouldn't be going to the bloody prom with sodding Julie Riggs!'

I thought for a moment. 'Maybe I should go talk to him.'

She looked repulsed by the idea.

I sighed. 'You *do like* him, don't you?'

As her cheeks were already red from crying, I couldn't tell if she was embarrassed by my question or not. 'Yes,' she eventually mumbled.

'Right. So, you can either talk to him yourself--'

'I can't do that!'

'--*or*,' I said over her, 'you can let *me* talk to him for you.'

It didn't take an idiot to see that Zen fancied Frankie. He was just better at hiding his feelings than she was. The main problem with him was that, unlike Frankie, he still seemed to be resisting the idea of the two of them together.

I led her back inside and left her to dry her eyes in the girls' toilets, while I went off in search of Zen.

I knew where he would be - his favourite place in the whole school: the music department. And, as expected, I found him perched on a piano stool, alone, in one of the spare practice rooms. He was strumming away on his dad's old guitar, which was encrusted with flower-power memorabilia stickers collected from endless pilgrimages and festivals.

I rapped on the door, even though it was already open and he could see me. 'Zen,' I said quietly over the soft lull of his playing. It had quite a nice sound to it, actually.

'I've been writing this for her,' he said without any encouragement, watching his own fingers carefully fly over the strings.

'For who?' I asked densely.

'Frankie.'

I listened for a little while longer.

'Look,' I eventually spoke. 'You know she fancies you. She's just not got a very good way of showing it, that's all.'

'I know.'

'And you *like* her, too.' I didn't need to question it; the fact that he was writing her a song was proof enough. He nodded in agreement, anyway.

'So, if you know she *likes* you, and you *like* her too, why don't you ask *her* out?'

He abruptly stopped his melodic playing.

'Because...'

'Because?' I pressed.

'Because I don't want to ruin our friendship, Loz,' he said without looking at me. 'We've known each other too long; we're so close. What if things didn't work out? What if afterwards we couldn't bear to be near each other--?'

'Whoa, whoa, Zen!' I stopped him. 'You guys have been friends for how long?'

He blinked at me.

'You clearly already know each other enough to know you want each other. What makes you think it wouldn't work out?' I frowned.

'Because sometimes it doesn't,' he replied matter-of-factly. Then he was silent as he looked meaningfully at me. 'Just like it didn't between...well, you and Dean.'

I felt my eyes widen in sheer disbelief; I hadn't expected *that*. Today really was a big day for revelations!

'I know what went on between you two, Loz.'

I turned away for a moment to collect myself. I bet Frankie had blabbed - I was going to bloody kill her the next time I saw her--!

'--I figured it out ages ago.' he assured me. 'And I'm sorry he hurt you in the end. If it helps, I won't tell anyone about it - not even Frankie. Though, at the moment, it doesn't seem like I'll be saying a whole lot to her for sometime. I bet she's pretty upset. I shouldn't have said anything, I know. I've made things a thousand times worse, but she really pushed me!...'

Zen's blasé attitude towards my relationship with Dean was unbelievable. I suddenly regretted not having confessed to him about it sooner. But then, he had known all along, anyway, and hadn't mentioned a thing about it. It clearly didn't make a blind bit of difference to him either way, whether I had fallen for another guy or not, and that did make me feel warm inside. Zen was far more mature than I gave him credit for, especially for a straight guy - he was a true friend.

'She is upset.' I nodded in answer to his concerns about Frankie, while still reeling from his admission. 'But more at how *she's* behaved, I'm guessing'

'Hmm.'

'Zen, just ask her out,' I sighed. 'Or at least ask her to prom.'

'Have you not been listening to a word I said?' he said tetchily.

'I have, and frankly, I think your doubts are unfounded.'

'I could *lose* her!'

'And what if you gain everything you could ever possibly want and more?' I added.

That made him think.

'Listen, I'm gonna leave you to it,' I said. 'But before I go, I just want to say this: you're more likely to lose her if you keep up this silly game of chase. If you really want her, don't push her away. Otherwise, one day, she just might not come back for more.'

A vague sense of déjà-vu at my own words sent a shiver up my spine. But I merely reminded myself not to dwell on darker times, and that, in mine and Dean's case, I had been right to push him away.

I left the room and Zen to a deadening silence. He needed time to weigh up his options. And in any case, I needed to entice Frankie out from her toilet sanctuary.

After convincing her that she really did need to get to her next lesson, I promised I would meet her right outside her Biology class when it finished and walk with her to the lunch.

'I can't believe you talked to him!' She shook her head at me as we barged our way past the bustling, starving crowd of students at 12:30pm.

'Would you rather I hadn't?'

She looked at me uncertainly for a second before muttering, 'no,' under her breath.

'He *does like* you, Frank. It had to be done.'

'Doesn't mean he's going to act on it, though,' she sulked.

We found a couple of spare seats at a table in the middle of the wide, airy dining hall, and unloaded our lunches.

As I tucked in, Frankie kept whipping her head round every which way, trying to locate Zen. 'Do you think he'll eat with us?'

'Why shouldn't he? He does most days you two argue,' I teased. Though I stopped joking when I caught sight of the murderous look in her eyes.

I honestly didn't see that there was anything to worry about, but that's not to say I didn't understand her anxieties. I had been there myself, once upon a time…'No! Don't go there, Loz!' I scolded myself.

At that precise moment, Zen appeared at the far entrance to the hall. I felt Frankie's body go rigid next to me. I turned to see that she had gone disturbingly pale, as well.

'Oh, God,' she whimpered.

Though I thought I knew better, for a moment there, I almost felt the same sense of trepidation she undoubtedly felt.

As he strode over to us, I noticed how grave his face was. When he reached our table, he stood in front of us and didn't bother pulling up a chair.

What was he going to say, I wondered? I looked from him to Frankie. They just stared expectantly at the other, their faces expressionless. But I sensed the emotional battle each was enduring inside.

Zen began. He cleared his throat and spoke shakily, 'Fr-Frankie?'

'Yes?' she answered edgily, eyes unwavering.

'W-will you…'

The hall suddenly started to quieten down. People from the surrounding tables, sensing something was up, started to turn round and look on nosily. I felt embarrassed for my friends.

'Will you…' I helped, getting uncomfortable, too.

'Will you,…' he repeated, his voice now audible throughout the large room, 'go to prom with…me?'

There was a muffled squeal somewhere in the background, and I managed to catch sight of a distraught-looking Julie Riggs scurrying out of the hall, hands to her face.

Ignoring this, and without a moment's hesitation, Frankie nodded and assented, 'Yes, I will!' Her responding smile was positively gleeful.

A round of applause broke out across the tables, hoots of congratulations and suggestive whistling filled the air. Zen exhaled deeply, smiling broadly, too, and then sat down.

'I am *so* embarrassed!' he murmured, the tips of his ears burning scarlet through his hair.

I smirked wickedly. 'I kinda feel sorry for Julie, though.'

But we all just fell about laughing at that, and resumed eating, carrying on acting as if nothing had even happened; like we pretty much did every time Zen and Frankie had a tiff.

CHAPTER 29.

Dean and his mum, Bonnie, had been renting a small flat in Norwich city centre for a few months, now.

Dean had enrolled at the city college, and was working hard to get his driving license as soon as possible. Once he could drive legally, he decided, he would hightail it out of there for good!

He still thought about Loz all the time. In truth, he had never got over him, not in all the time since that devastating night he and his mum had left The Brambles.

As expected, his mum hadn't taken it well, and had insisted on leaving the B&B immediately, while effing and blinding, saying how she had known all along that Dean wouldn't have been able to keep his perverted hands to himself. Apparently, she had hoped that confronting his "unnatural demons" in an environment where she could keep a closer eye on would do him the world of good. She had, of course, been very wrong.

And so, before he knew it, Dean's essentials were in the boot of his mum's second-hand Merc, and the two of them were whizzing up the roads as fast as the speed limit would allow.

John Price had been instructed to ship over their extra boxes once they had found themselves a place far enough away from "sinful temptation." John did as he was asked, despite thinking the whole thing was a massive overreaction.

Dean did feel sorry for him; he could tell John had real feelings for Bonnie. It was a comfort to know, at least, that Loz had an understanding, broadminded parent to turn to when he needed it. But for the sake of both his own and Loz's sanity, leaving had been only option. So Dean duly went along with his mum's, somewhat, insane plan of action.

These days, Dean no longer recognised himself. He was like an empty shell, completely soulless. His mother often spitefully commented on how much of a ghost he had become, haunting the flat. But if ever she missed John, Bonnie hid her feelings well enough. She had been transferred to the Norwich office of the same company she had worked for in Suffolk, and seemed to be ploughing through life happily, regardless. She still chose to ignore her son's blatant choice of lifestyle, though - ignorance was bliss, after all.

Dean's life wasn't as eventful, however. He didn't have many, if any, friends in Norwich, and the only thing that was keeping him going was knowing that his monthly salary packet from his weekend job at B&Q was bringing him one step closer to buying a car of his own. He would leave his mad mother far behind and go wherever the wind blew. But from there, there didn't seem to be much of a purpose left in life. He couldn't ever again imagine himself being able to feel the same sense of absolute love and contentedness he had once known, so what was the point in even trying? He deserved every ounce of pain he was dealt.

On one seemingly ordinary and uneventful day at the end of May, a brooding Dean lay awake in bed, unaware that something wonderful was about to happen. Today was the day that was going to change everything.

His mum was at work, and as he didn't have lessons until later that afternoon, he had decided to spend most of the day moping in bed in the drab-looking, crumbly-walled box room he had been allocated. It wasn't the nicest room in the flat by far, and he knew his mum had only given it to him as a form of punishment for his "sins." It didn't make any difference to Dean, either way, though. Being awake and being asleep were one in the same to him. All he ever seemed to do was dream about Loz, and it would only be when someone or something distracted him that he would come plummeting back down to Earth. Reality was too much of a depressing contrast, and it was enough to make him seriously consider the idea of finally ending it all for good, to allow himself to dream forevermore.

He did what he usually did when he was in one of gloomy moods, and stared up at the ceiling, counting the cracks. There were exactly ten, plus three large cobwebs, and he knew that - he had counted often enough - but it didn't stop him from recounting them over and over again in between visions of Loz's beautiful face.

'I'm losing the plot, here,' he thought unashamedly to himself

Just then, a buzzing noise came from the hard and dusty, wood-panelled floor below the bed, alerting him to a text message. This startled Dean a little, as he wasn't used to getting messages much anymore. He had all but lost contact with the friends he had made in Suffolk - mostly his own fault than theirs. He knew that if he still stayed friends with them, he wouldn't be able to stop himself from making every excuse to go down and visit them...and Loz.

He looked interestedly down at the impatiently flashing phone, and couldn't help but hope, even after so long, that it would be a kind word from Loz, maybe asking him to take him back.

Suddenly fuelled by that last shred of hope, Dean scooped up the phone, propped himself up in bed and scrolled earnestly down the little screen to find the message.

His heart sank spectacularly.

A horribly well-known number popped up on screen alongside the message:

I lied.

'*What*?!' Dean heard his voice escape from his lips. He thought about deleting it straightaway, but the adrenaline was now pumping fast in his veins. What did he mean by he had *lied*? If Alex had hoped this would catch his attention and plague him with curiosity, he was dead right!

Immediately, Dean threw back the covers and pressed the *call* button. He then commenced pacing around the room agitatedly.

Alex picked up on the first ring. 'Dean!'

'*What the fuck, Alex*?!'

'Okay, calm down.'

'Don't tell me to be calm! Just tell me exactly what you mean by you "lied!"'

'I'd rather tell you in person--'

'You're gonna tell me now!' Dean spat.

'Where are you...I can come and meet you today.'

'Alex!'

'Look, it'll take me two hours to get to Suffolk, tops--'

'I'm not in fucking Suffolk anymore, you dick!'

There was a pause on the line.

'Oh,' came Alex's rueful voice.

'Yes, "oh!"'

'So, where are you now, then?'

'None of your business!'

'Fine…So, does that mean you and…Loz aren't--'

'Nope! Not anymore - thanks to you!'

'…Dean, I'm so so--'

'Oh, the hell you are!'

'I am! I really, really, *truly* am. God, I so didn't mean for this to happen. It's just that, when you told me about you two, I,…I got so mad, and I wanted to make you pay, to make you understand--'

'Spare me your psychotic excuses! Just tell me what you meant in your bloody text! *Now!*'

'I'm getting to that!' Alex's tone quickly matched Dean's.

'Well, get there faster!'

'Dean, if you want to know exactly what happened, then you're going to have to be patient for a second and listen!'

Dean bit the inside of his cheek and inhaled deeply, holding back the fire in his belly. 'Okay, *fine!* Shoot.'

Alex sighed and carried on from where he left off. 'I was hurt, Dean. You'd gone away, forgotten about me and had chased after someone else--'

'Alex, that's not what--'

'--so, yes, I tried to get you pissed. I hoped that if you got so drunk that you forgot all about this *Loz*, then you'd come crawling back into my arms without any encouragement.

'It didn't go to plan, though. You confessed your undying love for him and collapsed unconscious in my arms, instead.'

Dean's heart hammered away.

'Nothing happened, Dean. I just lied and said it had, when, really, I was just jealous. I was jealous that Loz had managed to do the one thing I couldn't.'

'…What was that?' Dean's voice croaked.

'Win your heart.'

For a moment, Dean felt a pang of sympathy for his old friend. He really hadn't considered how much his relationship with Loz might have affected him, how deeply he must have felt about Dean.

'It was a bitter, twisted thing to do, lying to you like that, and it didn't take me long to realise that I had no right to mess with your relationship,' Alex then said. 'No matter how much it may hurt me, I suppose I could never stand in the way of love.'

Another brief pause followed. There was quite a lot for Dean to process. 'You know, you really should have told me this *a lot* sooner!' he eventually cried, voice breaking slightly and lost for anything else to say.

'Well, I tried to tell you before, but you wouldn't let me!'

'You should have tried to tell me everyday!'

'You wouldn't have heard it!'

'Can you blame me?'

Alex seemed to think for a moment. 'No, I guess not…Again, I am so sorry. I hope you can find it in your heart…'

But Dean wasn't really listening anymore. It had finally dawned on him. He hadn't betrayed Loz after all! 'Shit!' he laughed hysterically over Alex. 'What am I gonna do now?'

'Go get him back, I suppose,' Alex replied quietly after a moment.

Of course, it was so obvious! And no sooner had the suggestion been implanted in his head, than Dean had already thrown down the phone, rapidly changed clothes, scribbled a farewell note for his mum, and was out the door heading for the station.

'I'm coming back to you, Loz!' The voice in his head sang as his sprinted down the street.

CHAPTER 30.

The last school day before study leave was intense. School shirt signings took place, people cried, pranks on the teachers were played, and, of course, tonight was prom night!

Personally, I thought all the commotion was for nothing. Most of us would be back at the school's adjoining sixth form college next year, anyway. It was really only the layabouts who would be buggering off to pursue a lifelong career in benefit scrounging. Still, the prom bit was a pleasant idea; it would be nice to let my hair down for at least one night before I went back to being a studious hermit again for the next month or so.

My only problem was that, now Zen and Frankie were going to prom together, I had no-one to go with. They told me I could still tag along with them, but I knew I would only serve as a third wheel. Besides, it would have kind of defeated the object of them going as an official couple if I went with them. Poor Zen's efforts to woo Frankie would have all gone to waste, otherwise.

So I told them I was more than happy to go on alone. This wasn't strictly true, as I had once very much looked forward to the idea of going to prom with Dean, but now that that idea was shot to shit I wasn't about to spoil everyone else's fun. And anyway, I didn't need a partner in order to have a good time - whether or not it was with Dean. I was determined to make the most of the night, regardless.

Dad dropped me off outside the venue where the prom was being held in Bury town centre at 7:00pm, and the streets were lined with students from my year all dolled up for the occasion. Some people had really gone all out - guys in florescent-coloured suits, girls in billowing ball gowns, tiaras and feather boas. I suddenly felt underdressed, which was silly, because only a moment ago I had ludicrously got it into my head that *I* would be the overdressed one! I supposed it had something to do with not being used to wearing tuxes - it was certainly a luxury item of clothing for me.

My tux was a simple black number, complete with bow tie, that I had rented for a scorching price from a place in the town. Dad and Nana had insisted that I spoil myself and go for the waist coat and cravats etc., saying that prom was a once in a lifetime event. But I really only wanted the bare essentials; I knew they couldn't realistically afford to blow a fortune on something I would only be intending to wear for the one night.

'Hey…you look really smart tonight, mate.' Dad smiled at me as I went to open the door once he had managed to pull into one of the limited parking spaces on the roadside.

'Thanks,' I said quickly, hoping he wouldn't make an emotional scene in front of all my class peers.

'Your mum would have loved to see you like this.' His eyes twinkled.

Oh, God! Please, don't cry!

"Kay-I-love-you-bye!' And I sprung out of the car. 'Don't wait up - I'll get a taxi back,' I called into the rolled-down car window.

The weather tonight was lovely. The sun was just setting, the dusky, peach-coloured light illuminating the town horizon. It was a shame the event was being hosted indoors, really.

Despite the fine weather, I decided I would go straight inside to wait on the others. There may have been prom goers everywhere, but I didn't like the idea of the rest of the townsfolk gawping at me in my ensemble, especially while I was minus a significant other!

I passed the photographers in the foyer, deciding that a solo prom picture was definitely too sad, and went and found my place at our pre-booked table in the main function room. Zen and Frankie would know to find me there whenever they turned up.

As I studied the elegantly laid out table, I found that, unfortunately - though not surprisingly - alcohol was off the menu tonight. I also noticed I was among the very few people who were already seated - the ones, like me, who were glaringly single. Everyone else was all coupled up and queuing for souvenir photos. It was a desperately lonely feeling, but then at least I had that in common with the other rejects - we were all together in that sense.

The function room itself really was a spectacular sight. You couldn't see the ceiling for all the decorations that adorned it, and at the far end of the room there was also a stage, where the band and DJ were setting up. The events committee had truly outdone themselves this year, and the prospect of the night's events succeeded in lifting my mood ever so slightly.

About twenty minutes later, I was joined by a small group of people I didn't know very well. Seeing as there was only three in my little gang and the table seated seven, I had to accommodate others. Though, at the moment, it felt like *they* were accommodating *me* more than anything. They each gave me a smile and a nod in semi-recognition, but then huddled back together to prattle on about some random school gossip. I had never felt more awkward. They must have really thought me a loner.

It was getting late, now. Where were Zen and Frankie? I sent them each a text message.

8.30pm and dinner was served, while the jazz band played on in the background. Frankly, I couldn't wait for the disco to start. I mean, come on, a *jazz* band for an end of school prom? In the meantime, I was starving - for a change - and immediately tucked into my food. I had been idly playing with my cutlery and destroying my napkin in my boredom up until that point.

8:55pm. Still no Zen and Frankie. I rung them, but all I ever got was voicemail. I couldn't believe they *both* had their phones off! Needless to say, I was more than a little narked off by now. Didn't they realise it wasn't easy for me to be here all by myself? I may be putting on a brave face, but seeing everyone so couple-y and smug just reminded me all the more of what I didn't have: someone who loved me, someone who didn't care that they were with me and wanted the world to know it, and most of all, someone I trusted not to ever hurt me.

Except I had had all of that...once. The anguish that came with the memory was almost enough to make me want to cry into my food. But I told myself to get a grip, and concentrated on the bluesy music between mouthfuls of salmon fillet. Although I had never really tried wine before, I couldn't help but think, if somewhat depressingly, that a big glass of red would be entirely appropriate right about now.

It was about 9:26pm by the time Zen and Frankie did eventually show up, arms interlocked and smiling dreamily into one another. I knew the precise time, because I had been so bored, that all I could do was stare at my watch for the last half hour, while everyone else milled around me sociably. Even some of the supervising teachers - Mr Roth from R.E. and Miss Matheson from Biology - were getting into the swing of things, showing off their cringe-worthy moves on the dance floor.

'I've been messaging you two for ages - you've missed dinner!' I hissed when they slumped down beside me. 'Where the hell have you been, anyway?'

I was so relieved to see them, that I hadn't had time to take in how they looked. Zen had on something that his dad probably got married in, judging by the frayed sleeves and odd holes, and his hair was still an unruly mess as ever.

Frankie, in comparison, was a picture of loveliness in a stunning lilac, beaded gown that generously accentuated her curves - dare I say it, she even looked *feminine*? Her hair was made up high and decorated with butterfly clips, but already there were strands poking out. In fact, as I looked more closely, it was positively falling apart. Was I mistaken in thinking I saw I few twigs in there, as well? As I gazed a little closer at Zen, too, I noticed that he had faint, rose-pink lipstick marks on his collar and neck.

I raised an eyebrow at them both, but they just looked at me, and then smiled knowingly at each other. 'Actually, I don't think I want to know,' I sighed, throwing up my hands.

'We're sorry, hon. Honest we are.' Frankie batted her eyelashes guiltily at me.

'Yeah, well…it's your loss,' I sniffed, knowing full well that they hadn't really missed a lot.

A little while later, I wandered off in search of the toilets - they were back in the direction of the foyer. As I walked by the large, glass front doors, I cursorily looked out to see a few people lighting up cigarettes - mostly the trashy people. Among them, though, was Jammy.

Jammy hadn't, in all honesty, given me many, if any, problems since last year's incident. It was as if I no longer knew him anymore. But, naturally, I was still scared of him. My guess was that, even with Dean gone, he was still too embarrassed with himself about how he had attacked me, and worried that I might finally tattle on him if ever he provoked me again.

When his evil eyes flitted briefly in my direction, I hurriedly moved away, hoping he hadn't seen me. Being on the overly cautious side, I decided I didn't need the toilet all that badly after all, and went back into the main room - there was safety in numbers there.

By about 11:30pm, the prom king and queen had been declared (a predictably popular couple I had nothing to do with), and I had danced enough. I had grown tired of the excitable crowds, and so went off in search of fresh air. There was a little courtyard just outside the glazed double doors to the side of the stage.

White fairy lights clung to the trellises of the little balcony that led down onto the private patio. There weren't that many people outside, as most were indoors dancing to the cheesy disco tunes. All the noise had given me a bit of a headache, and the gentle breeze in the early summer night air felt good against my hot cheeks. As I looked up into the sky, I caught my breath. Millions of stars lit up the vast black ocean above, and for the first time in a long time, I felt quite at peace.

I must have been stood there for a good twenty minutes or so, because the next thing I knew, the final song of the night was being announced. The courtyard quickly emptied, with the exception of me. I watched on as couple after couple made their way back inside, hand in hand, all smiley and teary-eyed.

Between some of them - though not many - I could see that little glimmer of something. Something in the way their eyes locked and their bodies intertwined so naturally, as if they were an extension of each other. These were unmistakable signs of real love. The very type of love I had known.

I began to really miss Dean right about then. I also realised, to my amazement, that this was the first time in ages when I had properly allowed myself enough time and space to think freely. Though, of course, that invariably meant I thought about *him*. And at that moment, there were no other stresses to conveniently get in the way, which was *not* a good thing! My chest was already beginning to feel tense; a sign of worse to come if I kept this up, I was sure.

As I considered moving back inside, where the loudness of the music would hopefully drown out my thoughts, I became distracted by the heavy clomp of footsteps, which grew louder and louder as they came up close behind me.

'Loz?' a memorable voice resounded; the sound of which was like a lullaby. Though it stunned me, somewhat, my heart flying up into my mouth.

Dean?

I didn't need further confirmation than that, though. For just then, quite unexpectedly, something inside of me snapped. It hadn't taken much, but I knew I was done; I wouldn't be able to fool myself anymore. I no longer had the willpower to ignore him; it had been too long. I hadn't expected to bump into him tonight, but then I never thought I would ever hear from him again, anyway. I was instantly weakened. He had called me to him, and it was so tempting.

We were totally alone in each other's company. Though the choice of music in the background didn't help matters much, only ever encouraging my weakness. I just had to look at him, and I was ready to do that now, I decided; I had punished us both enough in that respect. And anyway, I could afford to acknowledge him and still hate him, I reasoned.

But, as I finally turned to face him, I knew that that would be virtually impossible.

'You look great.' His glistening eyes were wide and he sounded sincere.

'What do you want, Dean?' I muttered, trying, unsuccessfully, to act all defensive and as if his being here was neither a surprise nor of any significance.

Looking at him, I realised my memory of him hadn't done him enough justice; I was momentarily blinded. To anyone else, I thought, he might have looked rather tired and slightly dishevelled - even in a tux. But to my surrendered heart, he would always be a vision of perfection.

He carried on walking slowly towards me, arms stiff by his side, his eyes fixed on mine.

'I came to request the last dance,' he smiled weakly, eyes unblinking, 'with you.'

I gulped. I should have been back inside. Dean shouldn't have been here at all. But as I looked up at him, saw the way he saw me with such unwavering focus, such determination, I knew I would easily fold under his continuing burning gaze and become his to hold once more. The very last of my bullet proof defensive layers - the barrier wall I had been hiding behind to protect my heart - all but fell away, and I was the old me again, the incandescently happy me.

The music lulled gently around us, drawing us into each other. I was easily hypnotised by the young man in front of me. I hadn't realised how much I missed him, which, in itself, triggered memories of treasured moments together. It hurt, like a fresh razor being dragged right across my already mangled heart, when I was reminded of how long ago they were and how I had since survived. And yet, despite being the cause, Dean was the only cure I could think of. I was just so sick and tired of the endless pain; I could sense the quenchable relief and I thirsted after it. At that point in time, the mere steps between us felt like oceans apart.

He held out a trembling hand to me. 'May I?'

I propelled forward, took his hand in mine and revelled in their warmth and their worn, familiar grasp. By mere touch alone, I realised I was alive again, as I felt his warmness radiate through me until I was sure I was glowing. I heard him sigh in return, his eyes twitching, watching as he stroked my fingers. He then massaged them more meticulously, as if he knew he could or would not release me again. We danced in circles; no particular routine, just close - right where I wanted to be.

'You have no idea how long I've wanted to at least be able to do *this* again,' he breathed nervously, motioning at our clasped hands.

I smiled gently, but carried on staring into him, past his brilliant eyes and deep inside to the person within. I read his honest soul, really sensed the desperation that he had undoubtedly felt for so long, and I knew he yearned for me just as much as I did for him.

I freed my hand from his and stroked his cheek, feeling the light bristles of sporadic stubble. It was amazingly humbling. His eyes closed as he leant his face into my soothing hand.

'Loz, there's something I need--'

'Shh!' I silenced him. I wasn't going to let him spoil the moment. I had temporarily decided to forget about our previous antagonisms in the delirium of this sudden, yet wonderfully real, dream. He just glared back at me anxiously, but I took my hand off his shoulder and put a finger to his slightly chapped lips in finalisation before gently smoothing them with my thumb. He had no choice but to carry on dancing. Talk was for later.

I had completely lost myself in him. As I marvelled at his every flawless detail and his every gorgeous flaw, I was in danger of forgetting my own name, let alone everything else around me. This moment shouldn't end, I thought. It couldn't. The world could have crumbled right from beneath us and I wouldn't have feared, wouldn't have given it a second thought. Because we were together again, just like we were destined to be. Dead or alive, either way, we would still be lost in our own heaven.

∾

Simply by holding him again, Dean knew he was falling, if possible, even further under the dangerously drug-like addiction that was Laurence Price - the expression on his beatific face now so sure, so happy, when once, not too long ago, so enraged. Dean had hated having Loz feel that way about him; the evasive glances, the cold shoulders. It tore him up inside bitterly every time he even contemplated Loz in the very pain he, Dean, had inflicted on the single most important person in his life. But Loz was here in his arms, now, and Dean was so resolutely set on making sure that they would never stray far from each other's reach for as long as they both should breathe.

Dean became acutely aware of his, once thoroughly damaged, heart slowly repairing itself deep within him, from which he initially felt so sure he was beyond recovery. The emotional void was closing up. Every smile, every blink, every breath from Loz added yet another stitch to his wounds, and Dean couldn't help but beam at the deliciously instant gratification it gave him.

He had thought it vital to tell Loz the real truth. But, judging by the way he was around him now, Loz didn't seem to need it. Their current connection felt like a form of forgiveness in itself. It was as if Loz had finally triumphed over the tug of war battle in his mind over Dean's alleged past convictions and was resolved to move on with him, regardless. Just knowing this helped ease Dean's pained heart all the more.

One thing was for sure, though. Loz would have to find out the truth sooner or later…

CHAPTER 31.

The music began to die down. It was time to go, as the DJ announced his goodbyes to the crowd.

Realising that we would soon no longer be alone, I moved to break away from Dean's grip, only to find I couldn't. I turned back to see him slowly shaking his head. He knew what I was thinking.

'Does it matter?' he asked.

I supposed it didn't. It wasn't like either of us had much of a reputation to uphold anymore. So I left my hand comfortably placed in his, and smiled at him. Who really gave a damn about what anyone else thought, anyway?

He grinned in return and leant in, giving me a tentative peck on the cheek. I felt an almost electrical surge run straight through me. I hadn't realised how much I missed that feeling, how much I craved it.

People were starting to file outside, but hardly any of them looked twice at me and Dean. We merely stood there, awaiting judgement that never came. Everyone was too wrapped up in the emotions and excitement of the night to notice us. It was as if we were invisible.

'Wanna get out of here?' he eventually muttered, sensing we probably weren't going to be made social pariahs after all.

'Yeah.' I beamed. I didn't care where we went or what happened, so long as I was with him. 'Let me go tell the others first, though.'

He nodded in agreement and finally let me go.

Walking back inside, I saw the hall was slowly emptying. There were half-deflated balloons and confetti scattered across the open floor. High spirited prom couples escorted each other out the main doors at the far end, a few were crying together, and those who were still dotted around the round dinner tables were collecting their things and saying their goodbyes to neighbours and friends.

Zen and Frankie were at our table, looking impatient. They had been waiting for me.

Frankie scowled at me when she saw me, putting her hands on her hips matronly. 'Where the hell have you been?'

'Just outside getting some air.' I said unapologetically. 'You guys going?'

'We kind of have to. The place is closing,' Zen replied sardonically.

'Oh…Well, you two go on ahead. I'm just talking to someone at the moment. I'll get a taxi home later,' I lied.

'A taxi by yourself will cost a fortune!' said Zen.

'Oh, it won't be too much.'

'And *who* exactly have you been talking to?' Frankie asked suspiciously, getting to the point.

'Just someone I know,' I said truthfully.

'Oh?'

'Yeah.'

'Well, in that case…Frank, I'm gonna go ring my dad to come get us,' Zen declared, clearly already bored of my evasiveness. 'Can I borrow your phone?'

Frankie's curiosity, however, was untiring, as she continued eyeing me skeptically.

'Sure, here.' She thrust her phone at him and waited until he had disappeared out of earshot before turning to interrogate me further.

'Dean's here, isn't he.' It was more a statement than a question.

I just stared back at her, grinning, unabashed by her obvious disapproval.

'Loz, what he did--'

'What he did doesn't matter anymore.' My tone rung absolute and it surprised even me. It seemed as though I had already made up my mind about my future with Dean without even having consciously decided on anything. The more I began to think about it, though, the more I understood that I simply had to have him. Whatever he had done, it could be forgiven now. I had seen the unabated determination in his eyes and knew that I could learn to trust him again. He was solely devoted to me and no-one else.

'You know I think this is a very bad idea, hon,' she moaned.

'I know.' I just continued smiling defiantly at her. 'Thanks for your concern all the same, Frank.'

She massaged her temples in exasperation. 'Yeah, yeah. Well, I suppose you'd better get going, then, hadn't you? Mustn't keep the man waiting.'

I gave her a quick hug. 'Mustn't keep yours waiting, either.' I winked suggestively, quickly glancing in Zen's direction.

'Prank me when you get home. That's an order, Loz!' she said authoritatively, choosing to ignore my comment.

'Yes, ma'am.' I mockingly saluted, then ran back outside to where my destiny awaited me.

CHAPTER 32.

Pushing past the ingoing guests on my way back out onto the terrace, I spotted Dean straightaway. He was leaning over the balcony and gazing up into the sky, seemingly awe-stricken by the same starry sight as I had been when he had found me.

I smiled to myself, deciding to give him a moment. I knew facing me tonight would no doubt have been hard for him, not knowing how I would react to his sudden reappearance.

'It's nice, isn't it?' I eventually called out to him. A lot of people had filed back indoors, now. It wouldn't be long until we would be asked to leave the premises to make way for the cleaners.

He whirled round at the sound of my voice, the gleam of instant pleasure at seeing me again very much evident in his eyes. 'I thought you'd abandoned me,' he joked.

I stepped forward and chuckled. 'You'd have only tracked me down again, I'm sure.'

'I'd have tracked you to the edge of the Earth and beyond,' he said more quietly.

My lips began to fizz with a need much greater than desire to finally meet his.

'How did you know where to find me? How did you get here?' I blurted out instead, reminding myself that we weren't entirely alone.

The corners of his mouth curved upwards. 'I couldn't stand you up on prom night.' He then held up his arms and looked himself over. 'Your dad helped me out with something to wear for the occasion…'

It was only now that he had brought attention to it that I really saw. His whole outfit was ever so slightly too big for him; he had on his trainers, too, and the red, sun-bleached bow tie was all skew-whiff. If anything, though, he still looked adorable.

'My dad?'

He laughed. 'Yeah…it's kind of a loaner from him.' His tone then became abruptly serious. 'He, erm…he said to wish me luck… with *everything*.'

I giggled. '"Wink, wink," eh?'

He smiled, visibly relieved by my light-hearted response. 'Yeah,… just so.'

We both sighed.

'You know, I've really missed you,' he said gently, his eyes soft.

'I've missed you, too,' I answered just as honestly. I was too far beyond the point of denial, now.

In spite of the few people left milling around us, it felt as though we were in our own little bubble. We could have been standing talking in the middle of a noisy football stadium and, somehow, I don't think it would have ruined the intimacy of the moment.

'Where have you *been*?' I asked in a pained voice.

'Away…not too far…Norfolk, actually,' he mumbled.

I moved even closer to him, feeling entranced again by his mere presence.

'I still love you, Loz,' he mouthed. 'I could never stop,' he then added more audibly.

The next thing I knew, I had virtually flown the last few paces between us, and my face was now firmly locked onto his. He did not pull away. The familiar shape of his lips moulded easily into mine, moving together as if they had a mind of their own; as if they would never get enough. Whether anyone saw our shocking embrace, or made any snide remarks, I never noticed. I had completely given over every sense I had to Dean.

Dean was the first to finally break away. He chuckled amusedly as he caught his breath. I suddenly remembered I needed air, too!

His large hands caressed the side of my neck as he spoke. 'I guess we're not much of a secret anymore, then.'

I looked around to see at least eight people gawping at us. Not a sound was uttered between them. I turned my attention back to Dean and shrugged, completely unembarrassed. I honestly didn't give a rat's arse what anyone else thought, now. 'Oops,' I said with a devilish grin. '...But it doesn't matter, right?'

He flashed his teeth at me. 'Right.'

Out of the corner of my eye, I watched as some people tried, without success, to slip away unnoticed, desperate to pass on this new piece of scandalous gossip to anyone left inside who might listen.

Dean and I each tried to suppress another smirk.

Growing serious again, he then held my gaze. 'I need to tell you something, Loz. It...it's really important that you know,' he said. 'It's the whole reason why I even had the courage to come back here at all tonight. I hoped it would change everything...'

I didn't have a clue as to what he was talking about, but my interest was suddenly peeked. 'What's happened, Dean?' I asked uneasily.

'Well, you see...' he started. He then stopped, and his gaze shifted from me to behind me. His features became furious, the look in his eyes murderous.

I was a little scared to say the least. My hands were wrapped around his waist, and I tugged at the sides of his jacket in a weak attempt to snap him out of it. I didn't like his face like that. 'Dean?'

But his focus was still elsewhere, so I half-turned my neck to see what it was that had attracted his attention so.

Jammy.

He stepped out of the doorway and onto the little balcony.

'You!' Dean snarled at him.

I snapped round to face Dean again, suitably unnerved by Jammy's closeness. I tried to remember that I was safe with Dean beside me.

'Me,' Jammy agreed. I imagined the, no doubt icy, grin plastered across his long, horse-like face.

'Fuck off!' Dean spat.

'And miss you two going at it? As if!' he cackled. 'Who'd have thought, though, eh? Deano and Pricey.'

I was only now beginning to feel embarrassed by the remaining onlookers. I no longer wanted an audience.

'Go home, Jammy! Party's over!' Dean said angrily.

'Nah, nah. This is way too good to pass up!' he heckled. 'Oi, Ed, Johno! Come out here!'

I spun back round to see two of Jammy's wingmen, Eddy Collier and Jonathan Whitman, appear from inside. They were just as tall and broad as Jammy, with the same intimidating faces. From the look of their kinked noses, scarred cheeks and dented foreheads, you could tell they liked to play rough.

I tried to swallow back the huge lump of bile that had formed in my throat. Where were those teachers when you needed them?!

'Just leave us alone,' I whined, taking in the alarming size of the lads before us. Even if Dean could pack a punch, he definitely wasn't strong enough to fend off three brawny louts all on his own! It was kind of a given that I wouldn't be much use to anyone in combat.

Jammy just mimicked my tone and his pals howled with laughter.

'Watch it, *mate*!' Dean growled at him. He clung to my arm defensively.

Jammy strode over to us and I felt Dean's grip tighten. 'Or what, Deano? *What you gonna do?*'

The last of the people standing about us must have sensed something was sparking off, and had finally gone back inside out of the way. I hoped at least one of them had had the decency to fetch a teacher.

'Don't make me break your face, Jobson! Just leave us alone, alright?'

'Deano, the only thing you'll break is a nail, you *poof*!'

That made me snap. '"Poof?" Ha! That's rich coming from *you*!'

There was silence, and Jammy's face became a mixture of shock and irritation. Surely he didn't think this wouldn't have been brought up?

'You heard him, Jammy,' Dean added, seeming to appreciate my input. 'So unless you want to make the headlines tomorrow, I'd get going!'

'Oi, Jammy, what's them bum-boys getting at?' Eddy grunted behind him.

'Nothing, Ed,' he replied coolly, his expression now calculative. 'They're just spewing a load of shit. Sick *gay* shit.'

'You didn't seem to think it was so sick when you had your tongue wrapped around my tonsils!' I fired.

Then everything seemed to happen all at once. As Jammy went for me, Dean pushed me aside and lurched forward, punching him square in the stomach. Eddy and Johno weren't much use to their friend, however; they just stood there, mouths agape, apparently too stunned to move.

'You lying, twisted little faggot!' Jammy wheezed, now on his knees in front of Dean, clutching at his abdomen. 'As if I would!'

At that, Eddy and Johno seemed to regain some form of composure, and, taking heed of Jammy's last words, they then came at us full pelt.

'Go, Loz!' Dean hollered at me as he ducked away from Johno's swipes.

But I wasn't about to leave him stranded, if that's what he wanted. Besides, Eddy was already right up in my face. He had grabbed me by the scruff of my, once neatly pressed, shirt before I had even had the chance to consider dodging away from him.

'Hey! Watch the material, yeah?' I managed, though I was scared to death!

Eddy sniggered villainously. He then clenched his free hand and aimed to sock me in the mouth.

I pulled my lips tight together as if to create a shield over my teeth, and then squinted my eyes. Oh, God - this was going to hurt!

'No! Loz!' I heard Dean cry out helplessly.

In the knick of time, there came a loud, authoritative *Uh-hum*! Thank The Lord!

The hold on my shirt slackened ever so slightly, and I opened a cautious eye to see both Mr Roth and Miss Matheson standing by the open, glazed doors, arms folded.

'Having fun, boys?' Mr Roth demanded, storming over to untangle Johno and Dean, who had each other in a precariously tight headlock. I noticed Jammy was still gripping pathetically at his middle, standing a little to one side.

'Edward, let go of Laurence's shirt at once!' Miss Matheson barked.

Eddy did as he was told, and I was levitated back down to Earth.

'You will *all* be in exclusion for this tomorrow!' she sniffed. 'And your parents will also be informed--'

'But Miss!' I exclaimed.

'I don't want to hear it! I'm not interested in details right now. We will talk about it more--'

'But Miss, we've finished school,' Jammy interrupted her.

'Not until the exams are over, technically,' she insisted. 'So you'll all be coming in tomorrow, anyway. You can study in the exclusion room!'

'What's your name, son?' Mr Roth asked Dean.

'Dean Mackellar,' he said. 'I don't go to this school anymore, though, sir.'

'In which case, you're to leave the premises this instance!' Miss Matheson commanded.

I could feel myself begin to panic. I didn't want to be left alone with Jammy and his brutish mates – I would be killed!

'Not without Loz,' Dean said stubbornly.

A relieved smile crept back onto my face, and I could see the amount of disgust on Jammy's.

'Then you may wait out front,' she informed, coming over to escort me and the three burly baboons back inside.

'Honestly, boys! On prom night!' she tutted, giving me a shove in the small of my back.

'I'll wait in the foyer, Loz.' Dean called after me.

I breathed through the fit of nerves that threatened to surface. I hated getting told off, but I was even more scared of what was likely to become of me once the teachers' backs were turned!

After we were given our telling off, we were finally allowed to escape.

It was 1:00am, so I guess it wasn't all that surprising to see how empty the large room was. It was literally just us rowdy lot and the cleaners left behind.

As we were marched back through to the foyer, I felt lifted by the sight of Dean again. In spite of everything, knowing he would be with me in whatever happened next was a huge comfort.

We were instructed to go straight home, but as soon as the venue doors shut behind the teachers, Dean had grabbed a hold of my hand and we broke into a run, darting across the road.

I looked back over my shoulder to see Jammy and his friends a little way behind us, belting it after us. But Dean was fast, and I was being forced to run much faster than I had ever run before.

He dragged me down the cobbled hill and through the back streets in the vain hope, I guessed, of shaking them off.

'Where are we going?' I shouted breathlessly to him as he led me down a darkened, narrow alley.

Another check confirmed that we no longer seemed to be being followed.

'Dean, they're not there anymore.'

Just as I said that, however, and just as we were about to break through the opposite end of the long alleyway, two of our pursuers jumped out in front of us. I groaned at the sight of the taxi rank by the central car park that was within unbelievably easy reach. But the dark, imposing figures encroached upon us. They had beaten us to the punch.

'*Shit*!' Dean hissed as we skidded to a halt.

'There they are!' Jammy (unmistakably) roared.

We had no choice but to go back on ourselves. But by which point, our tormentors were already hot on our tails. It would be especially difficult to shake them off, now, given that we were growing increasingly tired.

Dean didn't seem to want to give up, though, and made to sprint with me in the opposite direction, anyway. If not his energy, his determination, at least, was inexhaustible.

But, as we were about to come out through the other side again, we met bully number three! Obviously having heard our fast, oncoming footsteps, Johno leapt out just in time for Dean and I to go crashing into his rock-solid body and then collapse back on ourselves onto the ground.

My head banged hard as it hit the gritted floor. '*Argh!*'

Wincing through the pain, I saw Dean beside me quickly raise himself up off of his front and onto his elbows. He looked reasonably unharmed as he hastily dusted the dirt from his too-long sleeves and attempted to get up.

I felt something warm pulsating at the back of my head, and I could smell a rather pungent rusty smell. I blinked a couple of times as my eyes struggled, for some reason, against their focus.

Dean turned to me, and I saw that his face had grown white with horror.

Three loud, though strangely indecipherable, voices echoed around me, and the next thing I heard was the frantic pounding of their footsteps as they sprinted off.

Dean was still there, though; he was already close beside me, but he seemed to be crying and muttering something fervently under his breath. He shook off his jacket, put it across his lap and gently lifted my head to rest it there.

He then whipped out his phone and dialled shakily. The sounds he was making into the receiver came out too quickly for me to understand, his mouth moving too fast. I did, however, manage to hear my name being mentioned every so often, but it was becoming harder to concentrate on things. I was starting to feel a little chilly, too.

As I lay there getting progressively colder, the pain simultaneously subsiding, I felt an enormous rush of tiredness envelop me. It was such a welcoming idea, sleep. I had never wanted to sleep more in all my life, and it felt as though it would be so easy, as if all I had to do was simply close my eyelids and that would be it.

'Loz!...Loz! *Please*, stay with me!...' Dean's momentarily clear voice broke through my incoherent haze.

I wanted to reach up to him, to dry his tear-stained cheeks, to let him know all would be okay. I was just so tired; he would understand.

'I love you,' I heard myself utter. But now I had to sleep.

My head lolled gently into his lap, and then I was gone.

EPILOGUE.

Forcing my eyes open took all the strength I could muster. It was as if they had been glued shut. The tiny slits of light that poked through blinded me.

I then became aware of a mild throbbing. Something pulled at my scalp. There was definitely something around my head.

'*Ow,*' I said croakily, and somewhat nasally.

I tried to lift my aching hand - which had a tube sticking out of it, wrapped under gauze - to feel around for the pain, but it was as if dumbbells had been attached to me. I only just about had the energy to squirm a little, to readjust my weighty limbs.

The light was getting easier to bear now; it wasn't quite so painful for my corneas. And as things gradually moved back into focus, I realised I wasn't anywhere I recognised.

It was a small, grey and white room, and I seemed to be propped up against something big and squashy - probably a pillow - while lying under a horrid pink blanket in a large, metal-railed bed. A small window ahead of me was shuttered off, and there was an acute beeping noise beside me. I would have turned to see what was going on, but I didn't want to aggravate my head, which still throbbed slightly.

I also felt that something was very wrong with my nose. I wriggled it a little, struck by the unfamiliar sensation. It felt like there was a stopper in it, and yet I was still perfectly able to breathe in and out. My hands didn't quite have the strength to explore this weird phenomenon just yet, however. Instead, I lay there and, without moving my head at all too much, glanced about me.

Even though it felt as though I had slept for a hundred years or more, I was still very tired. But the intrigue at my new surroundings prevented me from dropping off again.

The beeping noise was beginning to get on my nerves. It was incessant!

'Shut-up!' I moaned loudly, my voice clearer now - the sound was worse than my alarm clock!

Just then, the sheets around me ruffled involuntarily. I wasn't alone. I had disturbed something beside me, and it grappled across the bed towards me.

'Shhh. It's…okay, Loz. I'm here,' came a muffled, lazy, male voice.

'Where am I?' I asked out loud, unable to force myself to turn and look at the stranger.

Nothing.

'Hello?' I said.

Still nothing.

I felt around for something to shake for attention, and settled on a hand. But the touch of it was instantly recognisable.

My breathing became irregular. The beeping raced in response. 'Dean?' I gripped his hand tightly and shook it. 'Dean?'

Everything came back to me in a rush, and I realised at once that, of course, I was in a hospital room. It all made sense now, and I became so petrified by the sheer amount of things attached to me, that I dared not move again for fear that I would disrupt something that might have the power to turn me off for good!

'*Dean!*' I hissed.

'Um?' he grunted.

'*Wake up!*'

His voice suddenly rose excitedly and more coherently as he regained more consciousness. 'Loz?…Loz! You're awake!' He laughed, relieved. I could tell he was about to lean in and hug me then.

'Don't touch me!' I blurted out without thinking. I became very rigid. I didn't want him knocking out one of my many wires or tubes.

'Why not?' he asked, clearly offended.

'You might pull at something!'

Relieved again, he tittered at that. 'No, I won't!'

'What's happened to me, Dean?' I spluttered, near tears.

Sensing my rising hysteria, he shushed me, taking a hold of my one un-gauzed hand firmly in his own, and using his other hand to stroke my face. 'You cracked your head open, Loz; you lost a lot of blood.'

Oh, God! Did that make me brain damaged? I panicked as I tried to remember as many algebraic equations as possible. This wouldn't do! I had an exam in a week's time!…Or did I? How long had I been asleep?

'You're okay,' he assured, reading my anxiety-ridden face. 'You were out cold when they got you here, though. Thought I'd lost you for a minute, there,' he said quietly. 'But they've bandaged you up good. They were worried there might have been some further damage…' Oh, no! '…but I think you're fine. You've come around quite quickly, and you've remembered me, at least.' He smirked.

I gulped as I took all this in, picturing the turban-like headscarf I was undoubtedly wearing. I didn't honestly feel any different, except for maybe a little tender.

'Won't you look at me?' Dean asked timidly. 'It's okay to move, you know.'

I trusted him enough to do as he asked, ignoring any painful niggles at the back of my skull.

I almost cried at the sight of him; he was a right state - face unshaven, hair all ruffled and puffy-eyed. He looked as if he literally hadn't left my side all the time I had been unconscious.

I carelessly threw my arms around him, anyway, and hugged him to me.

'I'm just glad you're okay…I was so scared…' he mumbled softly into my shoulder as I nuzzled into him.

I eventually let him go and he sat himself back down on the chair he had pulled up next to the bed. He still kept a protective hand over mine, though.

'How long was I out for?' I asked, now more calm.

'You've been virtually comatose for two days,' he said gently.

Only two days. That didn't sound too bad.

'And Dad and Nana?'

'They've gone to get something to eat.'

I grimaced. So they *were* here.

'They'll be back soon,' he added.

I groaned. As much as I loved them and wanted to reassure them, I knew they would only fuss over me, and right now, Dean was the only one I wanted doing the fussing.

I then thought out loud, 'What about Zen and Frankie?'

I could just imagine the amount of angry and worried texts and messages left on my mobile.

'They're okay - they know. They've been to visit a couple of times,' he said. 'They left you a card' - He pointed over to the narrow, wheelie table that was pushed to the far side of the room, out of the way. Atop it was a pile of well wishers' cards - 'And some flowers… but the nurses took those away. Apparently, they were considered a health and safety risk to the other patients. Blah.'

'The killjoys!'

He smiled at me, the tired lines on his face becoming all the more visible.

'You're exhausted,' I confirmed.

He nodded. 'Yeah. I've only been able to grab a few winks here and there.'

'You didn't have to stay, you know.' Though, selfishly, I knew I didn't mean that.

He winked. 'I wouldn't have wanted to be anywhere else.'

I looked him over again and realised that he was actually still wearing items of clothing from prom. I looked down at myself and saw I was in one of those hideously unflattering mint-green hospital gowns.

'You haven't even changed!' I accused.

He shrugged. 'Didn't have much else to wear.'

'Smelly git.'

He snickered. 'Speak for yourself!'

'Uh, cheeky! I'm an invalid; I reserve the right to wallow in my own filth!'

He laughed. 'I should probably go get a nurse. They need to know you're awake.'

But he didn't attempt to go anywhere. I sensed that he wanted to savour this quiet moment with me. With no-one else around, we could truly be ourselves. It hadn't been like this in a long while.

'So what happens now?' I asked, ignoring his previous suggestion.

His brows creased into a hard line. 'You get better.'

'And then?' I pressed.

'…You finish your exams.'

He could be so frustrating sometimes. '*And then?*'

'Well, then you go on to sixth form and--'

'*Dean!*' I said impatiently. 'I meant between *us*. Where do *you* fit in?'

He thought about this. '…I guess that bit's up to you.'

'What? Why?'

His eyes closed and he sighed. 'Every time I'm near you, Loz, things just seem to go tits up. What with the whole Jammy fiasco, the,…the *break-up*' - He found that bit hard to say. I winced, too - 'And now prom!…I can't be any good for you…'

I suppose he was right to a certain extent. Ever since Dean had come into my world, my heart and soul had gone on one hell of a rollercoaster ride together. Sometimes I had the best time of my life, other times I just wanted to die. But all in all, I couldn't honestly say I would have done any of it differently. Not now that I finally had him back again, anyway. No matter how much he had hurt me, I couldn't deny the love I felt for him - it was far too strong to silence.

'Before you decide on anything, though, I have to tell you something--'

'Dean, there's nothing to decide on. I'm already--'

'Yes, I know, I know. But just hear me out,' he said firmly. 'I spoke to Alex a couple of days ago…'

I recoiled at his words, and an all too common achy feeling by my breast started up. I cursed that name!

He carried on quickly, seeing my discomfort. 'He called me to tell me the truth about what happened…in Luton that time.'

The *truth*? I felt my face scrunch up in confusion. It hurt to do it, too.

'We didn't sleep together, Loz,' he said simply.

My jaw dropped. '…What?'

'He only lied and said we had.'

I didn't know what to say; I really hadn't expected *this*. Dean just looked at me, waiting.

'You…didn't…sleep…with Alex?' I spluttered, still gaping at him. 'But, but why did he--?'

'Alex was apparently so jealous of you that, once I'd collapsed unconscious after our drinking session, he made up that vicious lie in the hope of splitting us up.'

I took in all of this and was suddenly livid. 'Well, tell him that, if it helps, it worked very well! The twat!'

Dean smirked. 'He knows that, and I've called him every vindictive name under the sun for it.'

I stared at him. 'And you *seriously* can't remember a thing from the rest of that night?'

He shook his head. 'Nope. And because I didn't know any better, I had little choice but to believe him when he said we'd…done stuff… together.'

'But what if he's lying *now*?' I said a little too sharply.

Dean shook his head again and spoke with such certainty this time, 'Trust me, Loz.'

And I did.

I thought for a moment. Something else still bothered me. 'You still shouldn't have lied to me about where you were going, Dean.'

'I know. I'm really sorry about that.' His eyes pleaded at me.

It took a minute to fully process everything. How was I supposed to react, now? I had spent months training myself to get over the vision of both him and Alex together, betraying me. Now, to know that it was all a scandalous falsehood concocted by this jealous ex-lover, to know that Dean had, in fact, been true to me all along…I suddenly felt guilty for having put him through so much, and, in turn, myself. It had all been completely unnecessary - a waste of time and tears. On the other hand, it *had* been all Alex's fault, and if ever I did meet him, I would definitely give him a piece of my mind!

I shoved the negative thoughts of Alex out of my mind and decided to concentrate on what really mattered: Dean and I. It was such a release knowing there was nothing to forgive anymore - no more skeletons in the closet.

I felt exhilarated, and smiled temptingly at Dean as I tugged at his arm, wanting to pull him onto the bed with me.

He complied, and wedged in awkwardly beside me, careful to leave me as much room as possible. I placed my arms back round him and kissed the top of his head lovingly.

'You're sure I won't pull out one of your tubes?' he teased, snuggling into me.

'M'eh, they probably aren't doing much, anyway.' I shrugged, hardly noticing they were there anymore.

We lay there for a little while, enjoying each other's comfort. This was the best medicine, for sure! I had all but forgotten the twinge at the back of my skull in all the excitement.

Then Dean spoke, 'You're amazing, you know that?'

I grinned to myself and sighed with mock arrogance, 'I know.'

'No, I mean it…you were *actually* going to forgive me. You were willing to love me, regardless of whether you knew the truth or not,' he said, looking up at me in sheer adoration.

I exhaled and admitted, 'It took me a long time to get to that point, Dean.'

'But you got there,' he encouraged.

'Yeah.' I nodded, then rested my chin on his head. '…I guess I couldn't keep on pretending.'

He lifted himself to kiss me tenderly on the lips; a tingling sensation spread through to every orifice of my body.

'I'm sorry for being so cold before,' I said meekly.

'I didn't blame you - I hated myself more than you can possibly know.' He went quiet, as if deep in thought. 'I hope you know that, in spite of all that's happened, I wouldn't…couldn't ever hurt you like that…*Ever!*'

I nodded. I didn't have to question it to know that that was true. 'I want us to move on from this together.'

'I think we can do that,' he agreed.

'No more secrets, though.'

'None.'

'Alright,' I said, attempting to readjust myself slightly. 'How are we going to make this work, then? I mean, you don't even live in Suffolk anymore.'

'I'll find somewhere. Maybe your dad will let me stay at the B&B - he's pretty cool. I can get a job to pay the rent and everything,' Dean said eagerly, sitting himself up more attentively.

'And school?'

'I can enrol at the local community college.'

'What about eventually going off to university?'

'We'll work something out. Maybe I won't even go.'

'What about your mum?' I asked.

'Sod her!'

'Dean.'

'What? She's a nutter!'

I laughed. 'Even so, she's still your mum.'

'I'm not going back to her, Loz,' he said adamantly. 'Ever since she was convinced I was going to hell, she's been making my life a *living* hell!'

'She'll come around.'

'Pffft, yeah right!'

I had to admit, it didn't seem likely; Bonnie Mackellar was very set in her ignorant ways. There were a lot of narrow-minded people out there, and Dean's mum was the cream of the crop.

'Besides,' he continued, while caressing my bandaged hand fondly with his roughened finger tips, 'so long as I have you, what do I need her for?'

I pulled him back into me and squeezed his shoulder tightly, my chest swollen with the love that welled up inside.

'You mean everything to me,' he whispered.

He meant everything to me, too.

'We'll make this work,' I promised him, blinking back new tears. 'Somehow, we *will!*'

Time then ceased to exist as we lay together as one, hearts in each other's hands. And that was how we would always stay; wanting each other...always.